Strategies for
Electronic Document and Health Record Management

Darice M. Grzybowski, MA, RHIA, FAHIMA

AHIMA-Approved ICD-10-CM/PCS Trainer

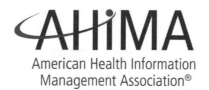

AHIMA
American Health Information
Management Association®

ISBN: **978-1-58426-199-5**
AHIMA Product No.: AB113013

AHIMA Staff:
Jessica Block, MA, Assistant Editor
Julie A. Dooling, RHIT, Technical Review
Jason O. Malley, Vice President, Business and Innovation
Ashley Latta, Production Development Editor
Lou Ann Wiedemann, MS, RHIA, FAHIMA, CDIP, CHDA, CPEHR, Technical Review
Pamela Woolf, Director of Publications

The websites listed in this book were current and valid as of the date of publication. However, webpage addresses and the information on them may change at any time. The user is encouraged to perform his or her own general web searches to locate any site addresses listed here that are no longer valid.

For more information about AHIMA Press publications, including updates, visit http://www.ahima.org/publications/updates.aspx.

American Health Information Management Association
233 North Michigan Avenue, 21st Floor
Chicago, Illinois 60601-5809
ahima.org

Contents

About the Author

Darice M. Grzybowski is a registered health information administrator (RHIA), fellow of the American Health Information Management Association (FAHIMA), and an AHIMA-approved ICD-10-CM/PCS trainer/ambassador. She has a bachelor of science degree from the University of Illinois and a master of arts degree with a focus on clinical data management from DePaul University School of New Learning. Other accomplishments include:

- Past president and two-time national delegate of the Illinois Health Information Management Association
- Advance Magazine's Top Ten HIM Professionals in 2010 Award Winner
- AHIMA Triumph Award Winner: Advancement in Computerization of Health Records
- ILHIMA and CAHIMA Distinguished Member Award Winner

Darice has over 30 years of experience in healthcare, including having worked as an HIM Regional Director, Consultant, National Industry Relations Manager for 3M Health Information Systems, and VP of Marketing for UK-based Craneware, Inc. Darice is an Adjunct Assistant Professor at the University of Illinois at Chicago's School of Biomedical and Health Information Sciences and, since 2005, President and Founder of H.I.Mentors, LLC, a best practice consulting, software, and strategic marketing firm. She has worked, researched, spoken, and written extensively on best practices in HIM, electronic health records and documentation management systems, revenue cycle, clinical documentation improvement, forms management, coding, computer-assisted coding, performance analytics, software development, and strategic marketing.

Acknowledgments

This book was written to provide strategic insight into the critical use of electronic document management systems (EDMS) in managing and maintaining the legal health record (LHR) for healthcare organizations. The content represents the culmination of over 20 years of experience in working with hospitals and physician practices that have struggled with electronic health record (EHR) systems that inadequately address the day-to-day working needs for improved workflow, labor productivity, documentation integrity, and patient privacy.

After 10 years of authoring an ongoing series of articles[1] focusing on EDMS and EHR considerations from the HIM perspective, the industry need for a book on this topic became clear to me from the continued feedback I have received. I was fortunate to be asked to author this publication and I am grateful to have had the opportunity to team up with the American Health Information Management Association to fill this knowledge gap.

There are a number of individuals and companies that I would like to recognize as contributors to this publication, and those who provided ongoing support and inspiration—and without whom I may not have completed this journey.

- ⊙ My family: Especially my parents, Sylvester C. Lulinski and Phyllis Lulinski, and son Jeffrey S. Grzybowski

- ⊙ Colleagues and contributors: W. Kelly McLendon (HIXperts), Deborah Kohn (Dak Systems Consulting), and Elaine Marmel (Marmel Enterprises, LLC)

- ⊙ My professional mentors and friends who motivated me throughout my career, particularly: Edward C. Stewart, Mary Mike Pavoni, Leslie A. Fox, Jennifer Cofer, Josh Pollatsek, Douglas Oblak, Ron Rowe, Jim Gravell, George Moon, Jody Ladwig, Keith Neilson, Gordon Craig, Cathy Hudspeth, Michele Ostrowski, and Kathleen M. Gallagher

- ⊙ Vendor contributors: McKesson Corporation, Chart Maxx—a division of Quest Diagnostics, Inc., Streamline Health, Inc.

I am also thankful to all the hard-working health information management (HIM) and information technology (IT) professionals, revenue cycle leaders, educators, and vendors who are my clients and who sought guidance on innovative and practice-oriented solutions as they tackled the transition from paper to hybrid to electronic health records. Congratulations to all those managers who have insisted on upholding best practice standards for record management by deploying fully functional EDMS solutions as a vital component of the EHR. By example, you have led the way for your colleagues, defended the rights of your patients in having quality documentation, and provided effective and efficient tools for your clinicians and staff.

---

[1] HCPro, Inc. (now Fortis); *Electronic Health Records Briefings 2005–2014*

This resource is dedicated with gratitude, to all of you and with a special note of thanks to my beloved aunt, godmother, personal physician, and role model—the late Dolores Lulinski-Dybalski, MD, who dedicated her life to practicing family medicine for 65 years and always upheld careful and complete documentation standards. She, and all of you, inspired me to enter into the health informatics field and achieve my highest potential by sharing knowledge with others.

My father used to always say that there is not enough time in life to make all of the mistakes yourself. This book is a perfect example of that truism. It will become the dog-eared reference on a nearby shelf for those of us in the healthcare industry involved in the challenging transition from paper to electronic health record automation.

The author and her collaborators, bringing years of field experience from working with scores of user installations and dozens of vendors, describe the issues, trade-offs, and decisions that must be made to effectively pull this off no matter where one stands during this evolution and the resulting hybrid environment.

This text sheds light on the conventional wisdom that does not appreciate the vast differences between EHR and EDMS systems. In the author's informative style, it carefully articulates the complicated (delicate) symbiotic relationship between the systems in the hybrid paper and electronic environments. A cornerstone to this differentiation is the episodic focus of this data set and the differences of post-discharge versus contemporaneous delivery of care.

Even sites enjoying the robustness of a Level 3 EDMS that is fully automated will glean from these lessons learned how to better leverage their own considerable investment and effort.

Right at the start, the introduction includes a "how to guide" for readers who represent the stakeholders associated with the legal record in the hybrid continuum environment of today. Throughout the text, the focus is on workflow and outcomes, not software features and functions.

This guide clearly helps the reader understand the difference between what we data geeks call persistence—the at-a-point-in-time paradigm of the legal record—versus the longitudinal clinical data perspective associated with an EHR system. This is neither a conflict nor a competition but reflects true synergy. The reader will see that these systems coexist because different trade-off decisions have to be made, a different workflow has to be supported and most importantly, a different goal has to be supported. That there are still both yellow pages and white pages in the phone book is an interesting example of the need for duality. One could always find all of the plumbers in the white pages; it would just take too long. The EDMS is designed, built, and implemented to support the legal health record.

To assist the reader on the journey, the author provides a plethora of tools to understand and create a document management strategy, framework, and roadmap through the transition. So as not to get lost, and to assist in knowing where to begin, a clear and concise hierarchy of the hybrid levels is presented.

Ms. Grzybowski shares her experience to educate the readers to avoid some of the most common and often ignored pitfalls, as well as providing best practice guidance and scenarios that find the proper balance among and between the trade-offs.

The result is that it becomes clear to the reader that the EDMS is the optimal system to support HIM workflow and to capture, manage, and provide access to the legal health record.

The author carefully details the importance of information governance for the reader. Health information management is the cornerstone for managing the legal health record. The electronic document management system is the catalyst for the integrity and timely, assured retrieval of health information management.

In order to ensure proper integrity throughout the lifecycle of this health information, the author describes often overlooked purge rules and criteria, retention standards, and the implications of legal documentation liability.

Another area of confusion brought into the light of day by the author is the underlying standards issues and conflicting opinions and guidance that must be dealt with by the industry. Standards, guidelines, laws, compliance, and regulatory requirements must all be consistently addressed. The well known quip attributed to my thesis advisor, Admiral (USN dec.) Grace Murray Hopper, is "the wonderful thing about standards is that there are so many of them to choose from." This book will help you not just choose, but understand the trade-offs.

The book also serves the reader as a resource guide. To maintain balance not often found in such a volume, the author conveniently points the reader to additional supporting material, both elsewhere in the book as well as the literature. Moreover, it provides FAQs, checklists, and exercises, making it both informative and educational. Also included are cookbook-style instructions for workflow documentation and design and universal best practice prototype designs.

The text also provides the organizational challenges including descriptions of the different roles and responsibilities of health information management in the new-world, automated environment.

Electronic health records may or may not have all of the capabilities that are needed. In a general sense, EDMSs must be a core system unless the functions and workflows articulated throughout this work regarding the legal health record are supported within the EHR. Enjoy the read and the road to effective electronic health information management.

Michael L. Glickman
President, Computer Network Architects, Inc.
Founding Member of Health Level (HL7) Working Group

Introduction

The purpose of this book is to provide a resource guide for healthcare facilities and health information managers who are considering or have already begun transitioning from paper medical records to electronic health records (EHRs). Clinicians, information technology experts, and health information management (HIM) professionals are experiencing challenges within hybrid record management environments. This challenge is particularly true when no adequate electronic document management system (EDMS) is in place as a component of the EHR, upon which the foundation of the legal health record (LHR) can be based.

This book is not intended as a technical guide or as a selection guide for choosing a specific vendor's solution. It is, however, intended to provide a deeper understanding as to how electronic document management systems function when utilized as a facility's legal health record, which is the suggested best practice discussed within this text. This book also intends to dispel myths and misunderstandings in the healthcare industry that assume that the need for document management software has been displaced by a discrete data-based EHR system. This false assumption typically stems from a lack of understanding of HIM workflow needs and thus this book is designed to provide details about the importance of using document management systems to support workflow efficiencies for healthcare organizations.

Health information managers, information technology managers, physicians, consultants, hospital executives, lawmakers, and other individuals and vendors that may design, sell, market, or otherwise work in the development of various health information and electronic health record systems may benefit from this book. As these individuals seek a way to manage the concerns presented by EHRs that include often inadequate workflow solutions, unacceptable printed output format, and difficult-to-manage release of information and fragmented file access, an understanding of innovation and best practices in the use of electronic document management systems is critical. To effectively provide information governance as an HIM professional, it is vital to have a strategy for document management that can provide a framework and roadmap to guide organizations through the transition to electronic health records. While this book is written primarily from the perspective of the needs of a hospital environment, many of the examples cited and recommended solutions can also apply to physician, alternative care, and post-discharge healthcare settings to serve as a guide for facilities to work toward achieving the most innovative best practices currently in place for electronic health record management.

This book draws heavily on the author's and various contributors' experiences working with hundreds of facilities across the United States over the past 30+ years; these facilities were in various stages of transition from the paper to the hybrid to the electronic health record environment. By sharing observations gathered as industry examples and presenting common sense best practices from the point of view of a professional health information manager, the journey to a more efficient and quality-focused electronic medical legal health record can be achieved.

⊙ How to Use This Book: Chapter Synopsis

This book will be helpful to individuals who are:

- ⊙ At any stage their journey to a fully electronic health record;
- ⊙ Considering multiple solutions and options in configuring their legal health record; and
- ⊙ Lacking resources to guide them through the process.

For these individuals, reading through the book from chapter 1 consecutively is recommended for the most thorough overview of electronic document management systems in a way that builds each concept upon information provided in the preceding chapter.

This book also will be of assistance to the experienced health information or technology manager or to facilities that began that transition from paper to electronic records a number of years ago, but have yet to move beyond the struggles of a complex hybrid environment to see recognizable benefit, improvement in productivity, or financial return on investment in their electronic health records systems. For these individuals, utilizing the book as a whole or by referencing specific topics will be viable options.

 Throughout the book, the following icon has been used in the margins to point out a key concept.

The following outline provides a brief description of chapter content:

Chapter 1 provides an overall understanding of electronic document management systems in healthcare by reviewing the roles an EDMS plays within the EHR. This chapter also provides an overview of the history of paper records and the evolution and definitions of hybrid records, as well as a comparison of scanning systems versus electronic document management systems, which typically are considered to contain a more sophisticated degree of workflow functionality within them. This chapter provides a way to create awareness, dispel industry myths or misperceptions, and educate stakeholders to various attributes and differences between the overall concept of an EHR and the EDMS.

Chapter 2 provides an in-depth background around workflow within an HIM department and how it can benefit from the use of a Level 3 electronic document management system. This chapter discusses the Master Patient Index, data integrity, deficiency management, and incomplete record processing.

Chapter 3 continues to review workflow for the HIM department within a combination EDMS and EHR environment for records management. While HIM-specific workflow is well understood within the HIM department, there is often a lack of understanding of the impact of these processes outside that department, and this chapter provides a basic understanding for those outside the HIM profession of more complex functions such as coding, grouping, data abstracting, clinical documentation improvement, release of information, and privacy issues.

Chapter 4 delves into the changing work environment of the EHR world. As with any technology, there are many facets to change management and human resources that are impacted by the adoption of EHR and EDMS, especially when using a poorly understood system like EDMS. This chapter provides examples of the changing job environment, stakeholder implications, and a myriad of other human resource topics related to EHR adoption and changing workflow throughout healthcare organizations.

Chapter 5 continues to discuss the human side of the EHR and related change management issues associated with EDMS implementation. This chapter focuses heavily on evolving job roles and work processes, the question of outsourcing of functions, staff productivity, and quality considerations within the HIM department particularly related to the prepping, scanning, and indexing functions, which are the key data capture points within an EDMS application.

Chapter 6 details the importance of forms management and forms inventory as part of the preparation for implementing an EHR and an EDMS. Proper forms management is the first step in assuring a solid implementation of any technology related to electronic record management. Unfortunately, forms management is frequently overlooked in the era of electronic documentation, usually being associated more with paper than online documentation; however having a solid forms strategy before, during, and after an EDMS implementation is equally, if not more, important than in the paper world.

Chapter 7 reviews the importance of recordkeeping for legal purposes, including the elusive legal health record inventory process. Record retention, archive, and purge issues do not disappear with electronic records and are actually more complex and often ignored in a digital environment. Preparing a record retention strategy is critical to success as facilities migrate and merge systems or tackle the challenges of a hybrid or fully electronic health record environment. As storage space become less expensive in a digital environment, record archive and destruction might be more about access and distribution issues; but actual retention and purging is worth reconsidering in light of the legal liability ramifications.

Chapter 8 discusses current issues in technical standards and organizational challenges related to adopting new technologies. There are often conflicting opinions relative to the strategies and growth of an electronic record system in healthcare. From equipment considerations to utilization of outsourcing vendors to assist with system selection, careful thought must be given to the expenditure of resources as the organization embraces automation for the legal health record.

Chapter 9 uses various case studies to provide a futuristic look at the importance of the centralized and virtual HIM departments through the use of electronic document management system technology. What was once viewed as only a bridge, technology is now being viewed more and more as a critical component of the electronic health record for long-term use to reduce the increasing labor demands for health information management staff in an industry plagued by a shortage of skilled technicians.

Chapter 10 provides a sampling of frequently asked questions about electronic document management systems to assist the reader when considering the adoption of EDMS technology within an EHR environment.

⊙ Disclaimer and Advice

This book is not intended as a substitute to facilities for legal guidance or for careful and deliberate investigation and review of any software solution portraying itself as an EHR or EDMS. Finally, the opinions and best practice advice is based on the author's experience and observations in working with several hundred healthcare organizations across the United States, as well as numerous published bibliographical resources pertaining to this topic, and is intended to serve as an industry resource for those seeking external expert guidance on the topic of EDMS for health information management purposes.

Understanding Electronic Health Record Management

As healthcare facilities transition patient medical records from paper to electronic records, a variety of challenging issues arise as part of electronic health record management (EHRM). EHRM encompasses both the overall *electronic health record* (EHR) environment, as well as specific software components such as the *electronic document management system* (EDMS). Understanding the evolution from paper to electronic health recordkeeping is helpful in analyzing current challenges and opportunities within the EHR and explains why the use of an EDMS is viewed as an essential component of the EHR for health information management (HIM) departments. The EDMS serves as a solution that successfully addresses HIM workflow and enables support of the legal health record (LHR). The glossary of terms in Appendix A will assist in navigating through the myriad of acronyms and abbreviations used here. The terms *chart, file, record,* or *health record* are all used interchangeably within this book to refer to a medical record. This chapter provides an introduction to EHRM by reviewing the history of paper record management as well as the assumptions and working models used to formulate theories in best practice and innovation in managing electronic medical records today.

⊙ Definition of the EDMS within the EHR

Electronic document management systems are complex software solutions that are somewhat synonymous with terms used within non-healthcare industries such as enterprise content management (ECM) or electronic record management (ERM). At the most basic level of definition, "an EDMS is a computer system consisting of many component technologies that enable healthcare businesses to use documents to realize significant improvements in work processes" (Kohn 2009).

Despite technology advancing at a rapid pace within the healthcare industry, a records management system needs to manage documents that originate and are kept in paper format as well as those that are digital in nature, and allow them to be accessible, and available to be archived, removed, or purged from the system. The system must be able to capture forms or documents that are:

- Generated from an electronic source and are then printed onto paper;
- Transmitted electronically from one system to another as part of the patient's legal medical record; and
- Originate as paper and must be scanned into the EDMS.

It is the primary premise of this book that the EDMS is still the optimal core solution and most innovative type of software today to support HIM workflow functions and provide access to the complete *legal* health record at a best practice level.

When discussing EDMS relative to the needs of healthcare facilities and health information management departments, an EDMS is intended to be used as the repository for replacing the paper-based medical record; and while it is not a substitute to the EHR's clinical environment supporting the creation of the documentation, the EDMS *is* a vital component of the EHR itself for maintaining and accessing the archived electronic legal health record. There are multiple ways in which documents are captured into an EDMS, including:

- Scanning paper forms such as consents, authorization forms, education sheets, or other documents that contain patient-specific clinical, demographic, or financial information.
- Faxed information such as admission orders, past radiology report results, physician referral notes, dictated report copies, or other documents that are received either in paper format and then scanned or received electronically and integrated directly into the EDMS without scanning.
- Computer output laser disk (COLD) feeds that are received electronically from other source systems. These feeds may include a report or formatted templates external to the healthcare organization, such as pathology reports, laboratory results, physician orders, nursing notes, rehabilitation summaries, and a myriad of other documents that upon transfer become a viewable part of the permanent legal health record housed within the EDMS.
- Health Level Seven (HL7) integration of messages and forms such as registration face sheets, provider-specific details concerning the identities of various caregivers, admission or discharge dates, and other data about the individual episode of care.
- Other forms and documents, regardless of electronic format, including alternate media such as photographs, telemetry strips, and even structured discrete data output.

However, the document capture component is only part of what makes the EDMS unique within an electronic health record (EHR) environment. The *key* differentiator of an EDMS used in a healthcare setting as compared to using only a scanning solution is the *workflow component*, which is specialized to the needs of managing medical records to comply with HIM practice standards. These practice standards with which healthcare facilities must comply are numerous and published primarily by the American Health Information Management Association (AHIMA) as well as various accrediting and standards organizations such as the Joint Commission and federal and state governmental regulations such as the Centers for Medicare and Medicaid Services (CMS). EDMS benefits have been described as "enhanced chart retrieval, electronic signature, workflow to manage chart completion, the ability to manage audits, and to serve as the centralized repository or legal archive" (Dooling and Downing 2011). See chapter 2 for examples of detailed workflow descriptions supported by the EDMS that are specifically tailored to accommodate operational aspects of medical record management.

⊙ Historical and Current Challenges of Paper Health Record Management

Before discussing the value of utilizing the EDMS as a vital component of the EHR in any detail, we need to step back and consider the history of paper medical records to understand how electronic document management systems evolved as a solution. Prior to the formal establishment of health information management (previously known as medical record administration) as a profession in 1928, medical records primarily consisted of index cards or a few paper notes, and only over time evolved into massive, movable file storage systems that contained large volumes of patient medical records. Also, in 1928, "the American College of Surgeons established the Association of Record Librarians of North America (ARLNA) and state this was done to 'elevate the standards of clinical records in hospitals and other medical institutions'"(AHIMA 2014). The ARLNA eventually became the American Medical Record Association (AMRA), and then was renamed the American Health Information Management Association (AHIMA) in the mid-1990s. But, regardless of name, this organization has always been the premier source of education-based practice standards for HIM professionals.

As the profession grew, so did the volume of accreditation or clinical care standards, documentation guidelines, laws, and other compliance and regulatory requirements that became the foundation of good recordkeeping. The practice standards and the software applications designed to accommodate those standards also continued to develop. See Appendix B for an sample of the AHIMA Practice Brief related to Managing the Transition from Paper to EHRs.

As a result of increasing complexity in medical care, technology, and compliance initiatives and the growth of medically related litigation, the sheer size or volume of the paper record also began to grow to accommodate the explosive growth in documentation content and number of forms. Paper files became thicker and multiple volumes of records quickly used up much of the space allotment in healthcare facilities. It was not uncommon to see medical records stacked in piles on cabinets, desks, in extra patient rooms, and disparate storage rooms throughout healthcare facilities, thus providing the physical motivation to optimize space utilization through use of software technologies.

Over time, additional media sources such as films, video recordings, audio recordings, photographs, computerized diagnostic equipment output, and monitoring strips were added as components of medical record documentation. These tools were adopted to capture additional information to supplement the existing narrative or data-based patient notes that were created as a result of a specific care encounter. However, the *paper* components of the medical record, typically stored within a paper file folder, became commonly known as the working medical record, and multiple challenges arose in this paper world to manage these documents.

Long-term storage of these medical records was labor, equipment, and space-intensive, as well as costly, and typically included:

- ⊙ On or offsite paper record storage in folders, boxes, cabinets, and on large stationary or movable file cabinets and shelves
- ⊙ Microfilm
- ⊙ Microfiche
- ⊙ Compact disks (individually or within a jukebox)

Aside from the cost of production and storage of microfiche, microfilm, and paper folders, these storage methods frequently utilized large and prime physical space within a healthcare facility. Accessing and using the records presented substantial challenges as well. Staff went through a multiple-step process to access the clinical information at remote sites if a medical record was needed for continuing patient care, release of information, studies, or audits. This searching function caused delays ranging from several hours to days to obtain the charts and information the reviewers needed. Simultaneous review by two or more individuals of a single record was impossible unless a physical duplicate of the record was provided. Thus the issue of managing the documents and the process or workflow surrounding these documents became a key industry need that had to be addressed if the electronic health record were to become a reality—and thus the evolution of the EDMS.

 The need to quickly and efficiently assemble disparate pieces of the medical record together, within a single episode of care, is still a critical need in healthcare today. This need to assemble disparate documents together from multiple systems, into a permanent, non-alterable single record, is met most easily and efficiently by use of an electronic document management system.

⊙ Hybrid Records

To understand how EDMS systems are currently used in healthcare facilities across the United States today, it is important to understand the evolution from the primarily paper environment described previously, to the hybrid state of recordkeeping that the majority of facilities use today. Hybrid medical record environments are most commonly thought of as a mix of paper and electronic medical record documentation. Electronic document management systems are frequently used as the fix to the hybrid environment as they present a way to manage all documents within a single episode of care, whether the source document is paper or electronic. However, a second breed of hybrid records has evolved: the mix of *scanned* electronic documents and electronic templates filled with discrete data elements in an electronic health record system or health information system. Neither hybrid system is a good solution for supporting workflow nor providing the infrastructure necessary to support a complete legal health record.

In some facilities, the EHR is devoid of the EDMS component altogether, and one may see a mix of some paper records still being kept as part of the LHR. Other systems may be fully dependent on trying to use the dynamic template-driven systems, and these types of systems are often called electronic health records. Other vendors or users may not view this type of electronic health record as a complete EHR, due to its lack of a static document management system component and would instead call those types of systems *longitudinal clinical record systems*. This mixture of content and format types within the various EHR-named systems can cause end user confusion due to the ever-evolving dynamic template content. The templates are updated based on the individual encounter and facility and may appear different at the time the record is actually accessed vs. how the data existed at the time the documentation was actually created during the specific episode of patient care. These scenarios can create a perception of lacking document integrity or validity in the medical record, which, in turn, can become a source of concern when considering legal accountability. It is easy to understand why there is industry confusion about this topic and why choosing which combination of electronic document and records management solutions is best for an environment can be difficult. This is especially true if the individuals guiding the EHR evolution have not previously worked in an environment that has overcome these challenges with the use of an EDMS.

The following scenarios will examine more detailed descriptions of common types of hybrid records that offer numerous challenges to the efficient management of health information and patient health records.

Scenario 1: Hybrid Record in a Partially-Paper, Partially-Electronic Environment

In this first scenario of a hybrid record, an organization may make the choice to retain its legal health record solely on paper, regardless of whether electronic or scanned documents already exist. In this case, various documents are stored on paper until the eventual designated time of destruction, even if they exist in the electronic system. As an alternative, documents might be created electronically, but printed onto paper, and the facility chooses to either scan these into an electronic system or archive them long term as an actual paper document, thus falling into this hybridization storage model. This hybrid environment results in two or more disparate locations in which to store and search for the legal health record, regardless of which system is being used to house the existing digital documents.

For example, a hospital may have all radiology reports online and electronically stored, except for Nuclear Medicine modality reports. As a result, the facility made a choice to keep all radiology final transcribed reports in their paper legal health record as opposed to declaring the electronic partially populated version as the source system. This fragmentation of storage described in Scenario 1, which is created by the mix of paper and electronic records, has been steadily increasing over time with the advancement of automated documentation systems and the increased use of scanning.

Scenario 2: Hybrid Record in a Fully Electronic Environment

In this scenario, all of the medical record elements may be captured and stored electronically for archival purposes, but scanned documents in the medical record are stored and accessed within data repositories that are separate from other electronically created and stored documents. The other electronic documentation within the clinical and electronic record system is typically more discrete in nature, often containing data elements or discrete clinical results that are field driven, as opposed to imaged documents. These are typically generated from various sources such as a laboratory system or a physician documentation or order entry system and are housed in other health information software or electronic health record software applications provided by one or more vendors.

This second hybrid environment creates functional limitations due to fragmentation of document storage within the episode of care. For example, instead of using a single access point for retrieval, cardiology results may be displayed and accessed from one function or repository, rehabilitation reports from another, and physician orders from still another repository such as the order entry system even though all the documents are fully electronic in format. Further complicating the situation is the fact that many of these types of hybrid electronic environments may not use any type of document management system as the legal health record; instead the environment relies on template-driven, discrete data elements viewed through customized or standardized templates that, on the surface, appear to serve as an electronic medical record.

Unfortunately, these systems are dynamic and rely on versioning often inaccessible to end users, degrading the integrity of the record to the end user who is trying to read or review the entire episode of care in a printable format. For example, an allergy may be recorded, but if later deleted from that field and updated, only the most recent change may display on a template as opposed to the original data and the corrected information that would be present on a document image that was properly amended. To amend items correctly, the original entry must be shown as well as the correction which identifies the person, date, and time the change was done. Printed formats depend on consistent viewable screens that provide stable, unchangeable content preservation and persistence, since this format is often required to be printed or electronically sent out to comply with court orders, subpoenas, and other release of information scenarios.

⊙ Implementation Variations of EDMS Models

There are three basic models that describe how document management systems or imaging systems are used and configured to try to accommodate hybrid records. Following is a brief description and diagram of each of these models.

A Level 1 EDMS Model

The diagram shown in figure 1.1 depicts this configuration for a Level 1 EDMS model. Level 1 EDMS can be accomplished by using the partial functionality of the document imaging or scanning functions within an EHR. There are multiple vendors who sell this scanning functionality primarily as an add-on and alternative EDMS solution to the more robust data-driven EHR vendor software application.

Level 1—or the most basic level of functionality—is sustained in a facility's EHRM when electronically produced documents are created and stored elsewhere within various components of the electronic health record, leaving only the scanned document images to be stored within the EDMS or scanning system. At that point, if a workflow-oriented EDMS is in place, it is not being optimized to its intended capacity of managing the encounter as a single episode of care.

Healthcare facilities that choose a Level 1 model of document management typically share the following characteristics:

- ⊙ A lack of understanding of the functional intended use and differences between a document imaging system and an electronic document management system

- ⊙ A focus on technology efficiency at the point of care (clinical data input) compared to managing the medical record both concurrently and retrospectively

- ⊙ An inadequate budget to provide for the integration and interface of the electronic documents created outside the EDMS

- ⊙ A lack of knowledge about the value of the workflow infrastructure within the EDMS software and the impact that workflow has on the HIM department's productivity and efficiency when the record is managed as a single encounter for each episode of care

Figure 1.1   Electronic document management system model, level 1

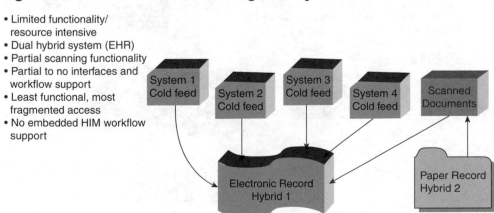

- Limited functionality/ resource intensive
- Dual hybrid system (EHR)
- Partial scanning functionality
- Partial to no interfaces and workflow support
- Least functional, most fragmented access
- No embedded HIM workflow support

A Level 2 EDMS Model

A growing number of healthcare facilities have recognized the need to unite all electronic documents with scanned documents into a single software environment. But, these facilities may not have fully adopted all of the workflow tools into operation, leaving a less than optimal configuration in place to support daily HIM responsibilities such as deficiency management, coding, and release of information.

Facilities that adopt a Level 2 configuration typically share these characteristics:

- ⊙ A less complex environment that does not require as much workflow support and specialization

- ⊙ A good understanding of the importance of unifying the documents of a single encounter as a replacement for the paper medical record

- ⊙ A single source health information systems solution in place with rudimentary workflow solutions in place for the HIM department

Figure 1.2 represents a Level 2 EDMS environment. A Level 2 configuration can be accommodated with a document-imaging or scanning solution—not a fully functional EDMS—which results in a less than optimal working environment due to the fragmentation of electronic documents now split between the scanning system and the electronic clinical information or documentation system. It also does not contain adequate workflow support for the HIM processing functions nor support for the LHR. It does provide for a relatively similar level of document capture and the ability to manage individual episodes of care for a single encounter without the fragmentation of record storage, and thus is still an improved model over a

Figure 1.2   Electronic document management system model, level 2

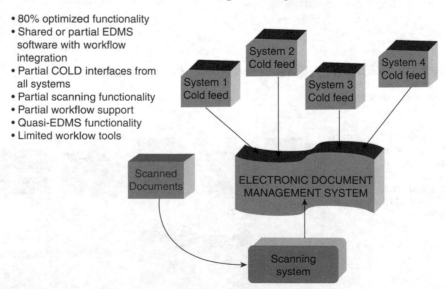

- 80% optimized functionality
- Shared or partial EDMS software with workflow integration
- Partial COLD interfaces from all systems
- Partial scanning functionality
- Partial workflow support
- Quasi-EDMS functionality
- Limited worklow tools

Level 1 system. The 80/20 rule was used as a way to illustrate a significant tipping point in volume at which point productivity tends to increase with automation.

A Level 3 EDMS Model

The most advanced configuration for an EDMS solution, and that which would be considered a best practice for health information managers, is one in which the *system includes workflow* and *infrastructure* support for the health information management department to manage the content, movement, and maintenance of the complete medical record.

In this model, all documents are united into a single repository as in Model 2, but the added level of workflow support provides advanced functionality to manage the record most effectively. The diagram shown in figure 1.3 delineates a Level 3 EDMS environment that includes full functionality and integration as a component of the electronic health record. This Level 3 solution requires a working interface between all electronic documents that may be created in any other source system, so that all documents are compiled as the complete permanent legal health record within the EDMS itself.

Facilities which utilize this type of model most typically share the following characteristics:

- ⊙ Involvement of HIM professionals in the design and roll-out of the electronic health record
- ⊙ A deeper understanding of workflow concepts for managing medical record information across a delivery system

Figure 1.3   Electronic document management system model, level 3

- 100% optimized functionality
- Dedicated EDMS software with workflow integration
- Full COLD interfaces from all systems
- Scanning functionality
- Reporting functionality
- Full legal health record support

Examples of COLD feeds

Laboratory Cold feed — Radiology Cold feed — Cardiology Cold feed — System 4 Cold feed

Scanned Documents → Electronic Document Management System

Master Patient Index | Release of Information | Coding and Abstracting | Deficiency Management

Workflow Tools

- ⊙ A focus on productivity and data integrity as it relates to the electronic health record
- ⊙ A thoroughly documented legal health record policy
- ⊙ A focus on efficiency and throughput standards from the health information management department

To help understand the practical application and critical need for a Level 3 EDMS for the HIM departments responsible for the facility's overall medical records, a comparison can be drawn from the evolution of radiology department film libraries. The transition from hard-copy film images to electronic image files and reports can provide a valuable lesson to health information managers on successfully replacing paper medical records with an effective EDMS application.

Large file rooms in radiology departments historically stored radiology films, reports, and other related documents. As picture archival communication systems (PACS) technology was implemented in facilities, the PACS software housed the complete episode of care for the radiology encounter in a single location, and the radiology departments were able to essentially replace the film library as full functionality of the legal health record. The PACS system stored both radiology reports plus films and was archived into a single electronic file for access and release of information requests. It is significant to note that even though the documents for PACS are housed *separately* from the EHR that may store other electronic clinical documents, and even though there may be a duplication between the original EHR-created documents and those integrated within the PACS system such as the dictated radiology report, the PACS system serves as the radiology department's replacement of the paper file. Both systems become valuable and irreplaceable components with the EHR to support radiology workflow and operations as well as the legal health record needs.

 Just as the PACS systems fully replaced the film libraries because they bring together the management of all types of radiological film studies across all modalities, the EDMS system with fully functional workflow serves as a best practice environment for HIM when the intent is to house the complete medical record in an electronic environment, regardless of the source of the electronic or paper document creation.

There is a common misperception in the industry that a Level 3 EDMS will add cost to the organization as opposed to a document scanning solution. While there is additional budgetary dollar investment that occurs upon the initial implementation of a Level 3 EDMS, the long-term efficiencies for workflow and the complete infrastructure to support the LHR would strategically justify the initial implementation cost. Instead, these facilities should be viewing the Level 3 investment as a dual stream of data—one that support the episodic-based legal health record and its related workflow, and one that provides longitudinal discrete data for ongoing template-driven reporting and comparisons.

The cost of each of these EDMS models generally increases incrementally with the improved functionality and requires more time to implement given the greater degree of integration in a Level 3 system as opposed to a Level 1 or

Level 2 system. However, hospitals typically experience long-term benefits such as increased productivity, improved turnaround time, and reduced expenses with greater investments in technology. With the expected connectivity and focus on quality as health information exchanges (HIEs) expand, the investment will be an area of focus in the future.

⊙ Document Scanning Systems Compared to Electronic Document Management Systems

In either of the Level 1 or Level 2 EDMS diagrams, the use of document imaging or scanning technologies are mentioned as an alternative to a workflow-based EDMS because they can be utilized for document capture. However, in a Level 3 EDMS, the workflow infrastructure provides the added support for a fully functional electronic document management system that *also* serves as the legal health record for release of information processes. Release of information describes the process where a request is received by an organization and a response is generated by providing a paper or electronic copy of an individual medical record episode within authorization and release legal guidelines specific to that facility, requestor, and type of record.

To clarify this point further, with document scanning systems such as Levels 1 and 2, the primary intent and use of the document scanning system is to replace and eliminate the need to store paper and provide a means of capturing digital images of the documents. In a Level 3 EDMS, in addition to the necessary component of document capture, the primary emphasis becomes managing those documents efficiently throughout the entire life cycle of the medical record within the workflow and system to focus on operational goals of the facility and the HIM department.

AHIMA's Document Imaging Toolkit states

> the most important reason for acquiring and implementing an (electronic) document management system is to capture and manage the organization's documents, not to (just) eliminate the paper. *Documents are (healthcare) organization assets.* Organizations must respect the necessity and strategic importance of managing its document assets just like the organization data, information, and cash assets (AHIMA 2012).

As HIM departments undergo transition from paper to hybrid to electronic records, facilities that have purchased standalone scanning solutions (as opposed to an EDMS solution that includes workflow) may incorrectly assume that they have all the components necessary to manage electronic medical records. These facilities might even be unaware of other options that improve functionality and ease of use of the system. This situation can worsen, because many similar-sounding or overlapping functionality components can appear within ancillary hospital information, revenue cycle, or electronic health record systems, but these systems might not provide the expected functionality. Industry vendors may inappropriately label or refer to scanning applications as electronic document management systems or refer to an EHR as a legal health record, leading to further confusion. As a result, healthcare facilities may currently be at a Level 1 or Level 2 EDMS model, yet they erroneously believe they are operating as a Level 3 EDMS.

The recognition that something is lacking in functionality has become apparent with user frustration being expressed more frequently for recent EHR systems that are proliferating in the industry. In the past few years, increasing concerns have been reported in the media related to the use of electronic health records and dissatisfaction of clinicians and administrators concerning the return on investment and even the potential inherent safety risks due to the poor documentation and operations of these systems. These concerns have been reported at both the hospital executive and the physician level as follows. According to recent poll results from the American College of Physicians and American EHR partners announced at the March 2013 Health Information Management System and Societies (HIMSS) meeting in New Orleans,

> 38% of respondents in 2012 said they wouldn't repurchase their EHR
> again compared to only one-quarter having this sentiment in 2010. The
> frustrations with EHRs grew somewhat along a range of measures from
> ease of use to the ability to lighten workloads (Nafziger 2013).

The 155-question survey was conducted with 10 professional societies and ran from March 2010 through December 2012, polling some 4,200 physicians to see how they felt about their certified EHRs' abilities to make them more productive or reach meaningful use objectives (Nafziger 2013).

The following chart provides an overview of the top EHR market trends based on a 2013 published article in the *Journal of AHIMA*, indicating changes over the past two years that show the most rapid growth of EHRs, all of which are non-EDMS-based solutions.

Vendor	Complete EHR	% Meaningful Use Attestation
Epic Systems	23,446	21.89%
Allscripts	12,741	11.90%
eClinicalWorks LLC	9,061	8.46%

Source: Richards 2013.

The situation hasn't gotten any better since the results above were published in 2013. For example, an article in the *Journal of AHIMA* states:

> The fact that some physicians are dissatisfied with EHRs was entirely
> predictable. There is still a lot of "shock and awe" among physicians
> who are alarmed by the disruptions to their workflow and the pace by
> which changes are happening. However, claims about EHR usability,
> configuration, workflow, and implementation were oversold to the provider
> community in many cases, and the reality is now settling in (Butler 2014).

Consideration of workflow needs as a driving strategy when selecting which tools are suited best to handle complex electronic health record documents and reevaluating electronic document management solutions as a core technology solution may positively shift the perception of automating clinical records for physicians and health information managers alike.

It should be noted that the remainder of this book will focus upon the Level 3 EDMS, as opposed to a Level 1 or Level 2 environment, as the best practice model being proposed to provide consistency in recommendations made and examples used throughout this publication. The advanced functionality of these systems makes the strategic adoption of a Level 3 EDMS a vital component of a successful EHR implementation. It is expected that the "EDMS will continue to be a bridge and support the EHR during this time of great change and transition" (Dooling and Downing 2011).

⊙ Best Practices and Innovation Takeaways

In summary, there are four main characteristics of a fully functional EDMS that differentiate it as a separate and vital component of the EHR within the EHRM environment. These include:

⊙ **Output as opposed to input focused:** While most electronic documents created at the point of care are clinician-input focused, the EDMS focuses on presenting a well formatted, permanent legal record that can be viewed electronically but printed onto paper copies for the release of information process that is typically required for court orders and subpoenas as well as other requests.

⊙ **Episodic as compared to longitudinally focused:** The intent of most EHRs is to collect data longitudinally for clinical comparison of results over time. The intent of the EDMS is to create a singular electronic file that houses all final documentation from a unique episode of care within the master patient index. Each unique file can then be referenced for historical chronological tracking and stand alone as a historical and legal record of care.

⊙ **Static persistent data as opposed to dynamic discrete data focused:** The medical record is dynamic all throughout its creation. Preliminary findings, report results, observations, and other documents are continually updated until final authentication and patient discharge. At the point when all documentation deficiencies are resolved, the record enters its permanent archive or filing state. The electronic archive is then in a stable state that does not change. In an EHR, the data continues to be dynamic and change, even after all information related to an episode of care is completed. For example, a medication list may continue to be updated with new medications. Without the patient providing information to update the older medication list, the medication list may appear altered upon the next admission, with incorrect assumptions made based on the changing information carrying over into a discrete data template. Persistent data, viewable as a document that cannot be altered after patient discharge, creates a reliable and integrity-based medical record for future access.

⊙ **Post-discharge status compared to current patient care status:** Most EHRs are designed with the clinician in mind and ways to make the data entry component of the medical record flow more easily. Little consideration is given to later retrieval of data, persistence of data, or printed format of data from a legal perspective. In a Level 3 EDMS, excellence in forms management practice comes into play. The EDMS focuses on the management of documents from a post-discharge status, where the record is more likely to be accessed for review of data exponentially more than in a current patient care status mode.

⊙ Best Practice Exercise

The following 12 questions may help identify if a facility is operating in a Level 1 or Level 2 EDMS environment and would benefit from the adoption or upgrade of an imaging system to a Level 3 EDMS. If there is a positive response to any of these questions, it may indicate functionality is below desired expectations and a review of the current document management process and structure should be considered.

1. Are you still maintaining any paper records (onsite or offsite storage) that were generated after you implemented your EHR or document management system?

2. Have you had to add any staff within the HIM department or other areas to assist with record processing, coding, release of information, data integrity, or other HIM-related functions after you implemented your EHR or document management system?

3. Do physicians or other clinicians need to sign on to complete documentation in more than one system?

4. If you have electronic records, are you able to process your release of information and audit requests internally, or are you relying on outsourced services to fulfill these requests?

5. Are you able to operate the majority of your HIM departmental functions off campus?

6. If subpoenaed for a printable copy of the medical record, would you be able to go to one source to print this?

7. Are you able to print only certain sections of the medical record upon request?

8. Are all documents in a single episode of care able to be locked down to prevent revision or updating once the record is complete?

9. Are electronic printed record formats consistent from an output perspective (compared to an input perspective) and standardized across patients?

10. Are bidirectional interfaces in place to assure changes in document content are reflected in all document storage locations?

11. Are 100 percent of all documents relative to a single episode of care available for chronological viewing through a single access point?

12. Are date range archives and purge functionality available for a complete episode or range of encounters?

To effectively manage the medical record on an encounter basis requires that one must be able to efficiently access, review, and archive an entire episode of care, from a single point of reference. The documentation must be gathered into a virtual electronic container so that it is accessible as a complete medical record. By the configuration of a Level 3 EDMS, the electronic medical record can chronologically tell the story of the patient from point of entry into the healthcare system to point of discharge.

REFERENCES

American Health Information Management Association. 2014. AHIMA & Our Work. http://www.ahima.org/about/history.aspx

American Health Information Management Association. 2012. AHIMA Document Management and Imaging Toolkit. Chicago: AHIMA.

Butler, M. 2014 (March). Healthcare reaches the EHR tipping point. *Journal of AHIMA* 85(3):25.

Dooling, J. and K. Downing. 2011 (October). Document management and imaging best practices to manage the hybrid record. *AHIMA Convention Proceedings.* Chicago: AHIMA.

Kohn, D. 2009 (March). How information technology supports virtual HIM departments. *Journal of AHIMA* 80(3): web extra. http://library.ahima.org/xpedio/groups/public/documents/ahima/bok1_043005.hcsp?dDocName=bok1_043005

Nafziger, B. 2013. Doc dissatisfaction with EHRs grows: Survey. DOTmed.com, Inc. http://www.dotmed.com/news/story/20637

Richards, B. 2013. EHR market share report shows top MU vendors. *Journal of AHIMA.* http://journal.ahima.org/2013/02/06/ehr-market-share-report-shows-top-mu-vendors/

Chapter 2

Health Information Management Workflow for Electronic Health Records and Document Management

Workflow is a generic term that is defined as the "progression of steps (tasks, events, interactions) that comprise a work process, involve two or more persons, and create or add value to the organization's activities" (WebFinance, Inc. 2014). However, when workflow is used in reference to an electronic health record (EHR) or electronic document management system (EDMS) intended for use with patient records, it also refers to the layer of application software that supports health information management (HIM) functionality. This chapter will provide the details necessary to explain how one would expect the unique workflow to be used or modified in a hybrid or all electronic record environments where an EDMS is in place. It also discusses some of the key functionality that typically is used within applications to support the tasks. Note that the terms *patient record, health record, medical record,* and *clinical record* may be used interchangeably throughout the text depending on the reference point.

⊙ Introduction to Workflow

Preparation time for implementation of an EDMS typically takes 6 to 18 months depending on the degree of readiness and the percentage of document automation within the healthcare facility, as well as how standardized the format of the documentation or forms may be. (See chapter 6 for a more detailed discussion of the process of forms management prior to an EDMS implementation.) During that preparatory time, it is critical to the success of the project to plan for changes within workflow for HIM. This is the time to examine the evolution from paper to hybrid to electronic recordkeeping infrastructure to most appropriately modify process steps to optimize benefits of the EHR and EDMS. This stage requires analysis and mapping of changes in the workflow process that will occur as the facility migrates to a more electronic environment.

The first step is to develop a process map that illustrates current steps in the procedure. The facility may choose to create a generic process map to illustrate the general workflow, or create individual flows for each major process within the HIM workflow, or both. The benefit of the *generic* workflow is that it can be used to help teach a wide variety of users of the system to understand how their role fits in to the overall HIM work process using an EDMS system. It also allows flexibility for minor changes in process, without the need to revise the primary workflow model. The benefit of the individual workflow diagrams is that they can be customized to fit very specific software and task applications variation within a facility. These maps become tools that are helpful for individual training around the processes prior to the implementation of a new system. Before deciding which approach might be most beneficial, consider the specific needs of the facility and the individuals who will need training, as well as the complexity and number of processes involved.

Use the following steps to create a workflow process map specific to the environment being studied—in this case the management of patient health records.

1. Observe current processes based on existing job descriptions. This should encompass all areas within the HIM department that touch the health record (whether it contains paper or electronic documents).

2. Observe current processes of the users of the health record who are external to the HIM department such as patient registration and access, billing, nursing, physicians, ancillary departments, external reviewers and auditors, and others.

3. Create a flow diagram of existing process.

4. Determine function-by-function changes that are necessary, both new and modified, as a result of EDMS adoption.

5. Review any expected changes in function on a task-by-task basis.

6. Create a new flow diagram of updated process changes and the new flow that will be in place post-EDMS adoption.

7. Update existing policies and procedures to prepare for training on new processes.

Figure 2.1 is a sample of a generic HIM workflow map that can be utilized in an EDMS environment. The sequence of the steps within this diagram is considered by the author to indicate a best practice model for the management of health records whether in paper, hybrid, or electronic environments and is reflective of an optimal number of steps in the process to maintain an efficient and effective workflow.

⊙ HIM Workflow Changes within an EDMS Environment

The discussion of HIM workflow changes within an EDMS environment in this chapter will cover the following functional areas for health information management professionals:

Figure 2.1 HIM workflow chart

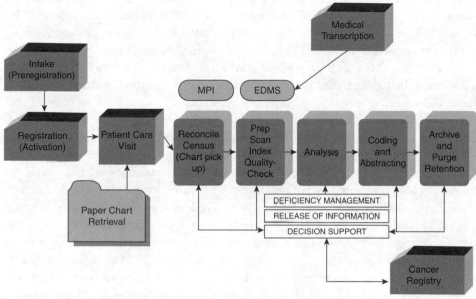

©Copyright 2011 H.I.Mentors—Confidential and to HIMentors, LLC and Client

- ⊙ Master patient index
- ⊙ Document and data integrity
- ⊙ Deficiency management and incomplete record processing

The following sections provide specific guidance on improving workflow for these core functions as a facility evolves in use of an EDMS, including discussion of examples of differences between traditional paper system workflow or within various hybrid environments. The individual work process elements will describe typical workflow considerations found in healthcare environments that are transitioning from paper to electronic records and the differences found in electronic workflow environments.

All examples demonstrate actual use cases as observed in the field, from healthcare providers who have utilized the EDMS as the legal health record component of the EHR. These sections provide a resource guide when identifying not only the changes in workflow from a current system to a future one, but in understanding functionality differences when evaluating EDMS software applications for implementation by a facility. Finally, these considerations are written to help identify the impact on the HIM department's medical record management function if using an EDMS instead of a generic EHR environment—one which does not contain a document management software component.

The Master Patient Index

A discussion about the master patient index (MPI) in a hospital cannot be completed without also talking about the topic of record integrity. Record integrity is made up of data integrity and document integrity. The two topics of the MPI and data integrity are closely related since the patient account or encounter number initiates the process of collecting the data throughout a patient's episode of care. Movement of the electronic medical record depends on access to an accurate account number, which is in turn linked to the medical record number, and then the actual documents. This section defines terms related to the MPI and discusses data and document integrity issues that may present challenges during the transition of paper to electronic records.

The MPI in a healthcare facility is a paper or electronic register that lists each patient or client episode of care within that facility and links it to a specific encounter number and, if existing, a unique organizational medical record number (MRN) or enterprise identification number. Throughout this book, you may see MRNs referred to as unit record numbers or patient identifiers. In contrast, encounter numbers are specific to a single visit, and sometimes referred to as episode numbers, account numbers, admissions, or visits. It is important to understand this concept, because, when discussing data integrity in terms of the legal health record, the reference point is from a single encounter or visit compared to all episodes of care longitudinally associated with the master patient index data of a patient. Data associated with the master patient index file commonly include patient demographics such as the name, contact information, primary physician of care, and basic patient demographics such as age, sex, and race. An enterprise medical record number is used to link visits of a patient between different entities in a healthcare system.

The MPI creates the underpinnings for accurate flow of information in a patient encounter so that the documents associated with that episode of care can be created, accessed, and stored as a complete electronic file of patient-specific documents, which then create the legal medical record. If an error exists within the MPI database—such as a duplicate medical record or account number—documents can become misfiled in a paper filing system or attached to an erroneous episode of care in an electronic system. This can create a potential risk to patient safety in that decisions made without full results can lead to the wrong diagnosis or orders being issued. This is true in both paper and electronic environments.

It is much more difficult to recognize a misplaced document if the entire contents of the medical record are not physically or electronically stored together, as is the case in EHRs that store scanned documents separately from other electronic created documents. Therefore, the use of an EDMS can assist in identifying these types of misplaced documents with a quality control process in place simply as a result of being the single point of access and location for all documents in the health record. Without appropriate quality controls in the MPI, which might include tools to prevent or identify duplication of medical record or account numbers, the future interoperability or data sharing between systems may be at risk, jeopardizing systems such as health information exchanges (HIEs) that are dependent on nonredundant and accurate data. Utilizing the EDMS environment to promote a clean MPI helps build quality controls to promote data integrity as patients move from one type of healthcare encounter such as diagnostic lab testing to another level of care like inpatient surgical admission.

The movement of the patient within a healthcare facility is associated with a simultaneous movement of the patient's medical record in a paper or electronic environment. Where a paper record exists, it is physically transferred with the patient by being hand-carried, mailed, or faxed to the next provider location. In an electronic environment, this movement occurs based on who has access rights to review the documentation, and access can be provided remotely and to multiple individuals simultaneously. To identify which electronic portion of the patient's medical record can be selected for movement, the MPI data is dependent on the accuracy of the information included for that patient relative to dates, physician names, patient names, and other identifying information, emphasizing once again the importance of quality control and data integrity in the MPI.

In an electronic environment, the software application within the master patient index shows the location of the activity of the patients at the visit level. There may be several different services provided to a patient during a single visit. Each visit begins with an encounter initiation date and time and ends with an encounter discharge date and time. A best practice in workflow is for the software system to visually display the visit detail within each encounter in a chronological sequence so that the end user can follow the chronology of the patient's visits and then retrieve the matching documents associated with that visit. The integrity of the MPI is maintained when the encounter listings are provided in reverse chronological order (most recent visit sequenced first). Multi-facility visits, such as to a physician's office, should only be viewed as part of the enterprise-wide MPI (eMPI) and not an individual facility's MPI to avoid fragmentation of the index. Zero charge accounts or canceled cases should not be a part of the MPI, although they may be referenced in a billing history or scheduling system.

Careful consideration should be given prior to using any type of series or recurring accounts that allow multiple episodes of documentation to be stored under a single number and, as a resulting convenience, billed as a single encounter across multiple dates. Series or recurring patient accounts should be used sparingly and only for repetitive identical therapies for a single and consistent set of therapeutic reasons. These types of accounts should never be used with multiple orders for different purposes within a single time and treatment period. In no circumstances should these types of accounts continue to exist if the episode of care is completed; otherwise, inadvertent charges and activities could be posted against an erroneous account and cause MPI errors. The admission and discharge dates should match the first date of service through the last date of visit. While some systems may automatically pre-register a monthly visit for a series patient account, the actual activation of the encounter should not occur in case the patient does not show up for the visit to avoid a false entry in the MPI that generates an invalid encounter with no charges. In series-type cases, an additional level of tracking to the specific service dates might become necessary to ensure complete documentation within an episode. This additional level of tracking is referred to as the utilization of check-in numbers when accounting for multiple visits within a single encounter number and is used to track the location of patient services within a single episode of care. For example, if a patient were registered as a lab patient, but also had a radiology diagnostic procedure and a visit to a facility on the same day, there may be distinct check-in numbers assigned under the master encounter number for that patient episode of care. All episodes of care are then matched to the medical record number, which is linked to the eMPI number, if one exists.

Patient registration functions, where the creation of the MPI occurs, are typically part of health information system (HIS) applications known as ADT (Admission/Discharge/Transfer) functionality. These functions carried over from the HIS environment to the electronic health record (EHR). In an EDMS system, the master patient index also serves a dual purpose as the reference index for the electronic document folders, to assure there is a repository for all existing documents to link together and form the comprehensive legal health record.

Document and Data Integrity

Record integrity processes ensure that both the data and documents within a paper or electronic medical record are as accurate and complete as possible. One of the primary roles of the HIM department, as the legal guardian of the medical record, is to provide data integrity processes that involve auditing the patient record and helping to design systems that promote accurate information in the medical record through completeness and timeliness reviews and audits.

While the generation of the medical record number and encounter or account number occur during the process of registering the patient to the healthcare facility, monitoring the accuracy of those numbers has historically been the responsibility of the health information management team because the integrity of these numbers within the patient record drives the use and access to the documents for future patient care, research, education, legal attestation, reimbursement, and many other uses. Monitoring of an encounter by encounter-based review is time consuming but can identify and provide an opportunity to merge paper or electronic records if a duplicate medical record or encounter number were to be discovered. Monitoring is the most common way that MPI duplications are identified. Increasingly, there are various software applications that can provide more sophisticated searches for duplication both at the time of patient registration and as a retrospective database scan to identify any missed duplication or errors. This type of MPI clean-up software is often used in MPI clean-up projects, which frequently occur in organizations that are switching to new MPI or health information system software or may be merging multiple facility MPIs together into an enterprise-wide system within an integrated delivery network (IDN) of healthcare facilities.

Data and documentation integrity issues related to the medical record can be varied. The upcoming sections provide some examples of the type of data and documentation errors that are commonly audited and tracked and need to be resolved within a paper or an EHR and EDMS environment from point of registration to point of scanning.

Duplicate Medical Record Numbers or Encounter Numbers

Duplicate MRNs or encounter numbers occur as the result of two or more identification numbers being assigned to the same patient. This might happen due to:

- ⊙ The lack of adequately checking demographic information carefully enough at the time of registration
- ⊙ Patient information being provided in error to the facility
- ⊙ Careless errors such as typos, name changes, and use of aliases

Correcting this situation often requires software to accommodate merges and separation of encounter data for the complete set of documentation within a single episode of care within the EDMS.

Inaccurate Admission and Discharge Dates or Times

Admission and discharge—the encounter start and the encounter end—dates and times need to reflect the actual date start and stop times when a patient is physically present. If the dates are not accurate, charges on the patient encounter may be placed inaccurately, insurance coverage may be denied, and turnaround time statistics may be incorrectly calculated; these are just a few examples of how poor data integrity may have a negative downstream impact. Specimen processing can utilize a *specimen received* and *results processed* as the start and end times. In this way, data integrity of documentation can be preserved when there are multiple encounters close in time to each other. Risk mitigation, timing of events, and the medico-legal aspect of tracking the timeline in patient care all benefit from accurate dates and times. EDMS software applications include clear identification of each episode and the related dates and times. This identification information is sometimes difficult to determine in an EHR environment without the EDMS software component as part of the EHR overall infrastructure since documents may be more longitudinally focused in the EHR than in the EDMS.

Missing Documents

Each order within the medical record is intended to produce a piece of documentation content—potentially a unique document—at the conclusion or fulfillment of that order. For example:

- ⊙ If a patient consultation is ordered by the attending physician, the consultant must provide a consultation note.
- ⊙ If an electrocardiogram or a complete blood count laboratory test is ordered, when the exam or test is completed, the results must be visibly documented.
- ⊙ If a patient is to have blood pressure monitored every hour, there needs to be a documented note as to the result of that monitoring.
- ⊙ If the order entry system contains orders that are not fulfilled, and results are not present that match the orders, this must be reconciled.

The EDMS provides a single environment from which to review and resolve any documentation discrepancies to assist with completion and compliance.

Documents that Are Mislabeled, Stamped, or Created with an Erroneous Number

The situation of mislabeling, stamping, or creating documents with a wrong number can happen in both the paper and electronic environments. As paper documents are received, they are prepped for processing by sorting them in a certain order and examining them for physical problems such as ripped pages or staples that may disrupt the scanning. During the prepping process with the use of an EDMS, other paper document errors are likely to be discovered since the prepping phase closely examines any received paper documents at the start of the record processing phase. However, if there is no scanning process involved and documents are created in electronic format only, yet appended to the wrong electronic medical record file within the MPI, it is less likely that software alone can uncover these errors unless found accidentally when reviewing the electronic chart.

Illegible or Blurred Documents

Documents may get scanned into the system with various flaws—they might be too dark, from colored paper, taped, stapled, and so on; or a problem might be created due to the electronic transfer or the scan itself. The need to recreate, flag, or clarify the content on documents can be done within the EDMS application by removing or replacing or editing such documents and rescanning (if needed) to eliminate these problems.

Data Corrections, Retractions, and Amendments

In an EDMS environment, if there is a correction made to the document—for example, to rectify the incorrect spelling of a patient name—usually only the corrected document becomes visible in the EDMS view, though the previous version of the document might be available. Retractions are changes to documentation after the fact, not necessarily due to an error, but potentially due to an edit. Amendments involve additional information or clarification of information from either the provider or the patient to be attached to the record. Policies and procedures at the facility level must guide policy to ensure these changes are handled properly. It is critical to note that the EDMS workflow software must support this process and data trail within the legal health record.

Data Reassignments

Data reassignments, also referred to as overlays, occur when documents are assigned either to an incorrect encounter number for the same patient or to an entirely separate patient either through erroneously scanned document placement or errant computer output laser disk (COLD) feed to a wrong encounter. The presence of clinical results attached to the wrong patient may cause erroneous medical treatment and clinical decision making. Both situations are dangerous to patient care and must be corrected immediately if and when identified. The EDMS workflow application must allow removal of documentation from the incorrect episode of care, and placement in the correct episode of care, within the correct sequence of forms.

Data Resequencing

The ability to sequence documentation within a complete episode of care—for example, chronologically by document type or in date order—is an essential feature of EDMS workflow software. Resequencing that data if a document were to have erroneous information is also an important feature of an EDMS system, so that references to these episodes of care maintain their chronological integrity. If a document were to appear out of order, have an incorrect date assigned to it, or arrive after the bulk of documentation is received, such as in the case of late or loose reports, errors, or omissions in accessing the data for release of information might result. Therefore, this feature must be accommodated by the EHR or EDMS software so as to maintain the integrity of the record. Simply appending the late information to the back of the record would cause confusion to the end user reviewing the information and might be easily skipped in retrieval processes.

Inaccurate Census Status

An increasing data integrity issue seen in facilities today is the inaccurate census status such as identifying a patient within a wrong care type upon discharge. For example, consider the patient who is treated as an inpatient, with an order for inpatient admission, but retrospectively (post-discharge) is changed into an observation status for census and billing purposes. In rare cases this may be legitimately done because of an error. However, more frequently this may be done due to the patient not meeting certain criteria for admission or severity or payor guidelines. Retrospective changes in this data element can create severe problems throughout the information system. For example, different guidelines exist based on the census status of a patient including utilization of care criteria, documentation requirements for the medical staff, and differing coding and grouping rules when processing the health record for insurance purposes. If an incorrect status is used, a patient may be discharged from a facility too early, a physician may not complete the documentation fully, hospital discharge statistics may be incorrectly calculated and insurance coverage may even be denied. Regardless of the policy and process that guide these types of errors, the EDMS must provide a clear audit trail to categorize the complete encounter of care and to ensure no fragment of documentation is missed.

Missing Records

When the entire medical record is delayed or missing, an incident report should be prepared that records any gaps in time in which the transfer from active patient care by clinicians to retrospective processing by the HIM. Documentation should be completed concurrently—that is, at the end of shift—in patient care encounters to guarantee transition of communication issues between practitioners. When gaps occur in documentation, the risk of error increases. The EDMS can be used as a vital tool for monitoring completeness of received records.

Consider carefully this last scenario of how facilities manage missing records. In the 100 percent paper environment of medical recordkeeping, daily discharge reconciliation is the process of ensuring that all records are collected for patients who are discharged from the facility. After collection, they are reviewed for completeness. This process is referred to as record reconciliation and involves reconciliation between a discharge encounter list and the actual physical receipt of the record. Where there are still portions of paper records being generated or printed, collection of even a portion of the chart should occur and go through paper reconciliation. However, if no paper output of records exists, consideration must be given to an alternative process of record reconciliation to ensure completeness within the EHR itself. This alternate process requires generating an electronic list that displays total output of documents (including number and type) from any electronic system feeding into the EHR and comparing that list to a list of total input of received documents entering into the EDMS. This comparison process of reconciliation of electronic files should be a vital component of any EHR or EDMS. Unfortunately, this step is commonly skipped in electronic environments, and often not identified as a problem until late in the process of searching for a missing record or documents. A problem that some facilities experience which they use to explain "missing" encounters from a facility is not a problem with missing documentation at all. It is a problem that occurs when a patient registration is activated and an encounter number assigned when there was no actual patient visit. These are sometimes referred to as "zero charge" cases. They most frequently occur when a registration is completed automatically on an assumption of a returned visit to a facility, or in cases where someone is pre-registered for care and the case is activated prior to the patient actually appearing for the visit. A cancelation occurs, but the encounter number has already been created.

The EDMS can assist in identifying these cases because a scanned document can be attached to the encounter, along with any paperwork that has already been completed, with a note stating "Encounter number of xx-xx-xxxx date has been canceled." Automation could also be accomplished via software products that can identify these zero cases and delete them from the MPI so that they do not appear accessible to end users. In this way, there is no mistaken care provided or erroneous coding or billing done that demand unnecessary work on these cases. Best practices in this area dictate that registrations should not be automatically activated; instead, wait until the individual is physically present to receive services. Following best practices in this area avoids creating false census entries into an MPI.

The recommended electronic reconciliation process referred to previously that can exist in the electronic workflow component of an EDMS is for *specific form content*. It is both an input and output balancing procedure. This process guarantees that there is still a checkpoint at which all charts that *should* be electronically received for an encounter have *actually been received* within the application. For example, if a radiology department provides services to 50 patients in a day, there should be 50 encounters with separate and unique account numbers and associated documentation content within the electronic folder in the EDMS, regardless of how many individual examinations are provided per patient. The source systems that provide the COLD feeds into an EDMS should be reconciled between that which was sent, and that which was received. Any variations to this count that create an imbalance should then force an alert so that the situation can be investigated and resolved. This is something that is not possible in an EHR that does not use an EDMS because of the difficulty in tracking the disparate information.

The importance of viewing the medical record as a whole, which can be done effectively within the Level 3 EDMS model, becomes increasingly critical for quality control for the facility. Identification of any of the aforementioned data integrity issues can be extremely difficult and time consuming in a fragmented model (Level 1) where users have to access reports from different source document locations outside an EDMS. Problems might not be discovered or there may be inadequate staff to perform the audits since the time to go in and out of different data sources to retrieve various documents and reports can take considerably longer than viewing a document within an EDMS.

To illustrate this point further, a recently observed hospital system has attempted to operate in an environment without having in place an EDMS as their primary legal health record. This HIM department has gradually added over 20 full-time staff members within the HIM department to provide ongoing monitoring and support across three hospitals to handle the quantity of data integrity problems that have occurred since the implementation of their core EHR due to the lack of the EDMS. The time it takes to review and correct what would be a routine number of data integrity errors or issues becomes increasingly extended without the assistance of EDMS tools for episodic MPI and data integrity control. While these topics do not include *every* potential data integrity issue, they serve as a reminder of the importance of data control with HIM workflow to maintain the quality and usefulness of the electronic health record.

Therefore, the case for utilizing the EDMS as the legal health record (LHR) within the EHR starts with the very creation point of the MPI and with the first documents inserted or received into the medical record.

Deficiency Management and Incomplete Record Processing

Deficiency management and incomplete record processing are core workflow components of the discharged patient medical record within the HIM department. As deficiencies are identified, the paper or electronic record is maintained in an incomplete state. The identification of typical deficiency processing and the steps needed to resolve those deficiencies and complete the medical record are described in detail in this section, along with tips on how to best handle deficiency processing within an electronic environment. Deficiency management refers to the process of auditing the content in the documents of the record to ensure the documentation is as complete as should be as based on the internal standards of the facility and any accreditation or state and federal regulatory standards that may be in place. The intent of this book is not to review or list those standards of deficiency identification, but rather to recognize that a variety of these standards exist, and that flexibility in the workflow for this task is an important process in health information management that should be accommodated. The EDMS system workflow provides specialized tools that can assist the facility in performing this process efficiently and effectively. The following tasks are examples of deficiency management within an EDMS environment.

Deficiency Analysis

Deficiency analysis represents the auditing process whereby the records are analyzed for elements that may be missing and cause the record to be incomplete or deficient in content. The degree of completeness is defined at the facility level by a combination of internal policy and procedure and external accreditation and regulatory standards. Some facilities choose to forego the analysis process altogether on certain types of charts and other facilities review the complete record. The elements of completion may vary and the EDMS deficiency workflow solution should be able to handle the complete spectrum of deficiency analysis across all patient types, clinicians, settings, and document types. Integration of the deficiency system with the dictation and transcription system is an essential key to ensure seamless and automatic deficiency flagging, automatic pending hold to completion, and automatic completion in this workflow.

By using an EDMS to house the complete medical record, all of the documents viewed and flagged for incomplete notation in the deficiency analysis process can be sequenced similarly to sections within a paper chart. Reviewing a paper chart might result in a deficient item such as a missing dictation of a specific operative report being flagged for completion. A missing document can be flagged in the EDMS workflow software that assists in the management of deficiencies until the point in time when the record becomes complete.

 When a record in an EDMS system is determined to be complete, the only changes made after that time are treated as addendums to the documentation in the chart. Since an EHR is dynamic in nature when compared to an EDMS, the EHR may have changing versions of screen-viewable content in certain documents, even after the record may be deemed complete by definition of the facility and medical staff. These differing versions of screen-viewable content are problematic from a data integrity, legal, and stability perspective of retrospective review.

All deficiency analysis requires a method of communication to clinicians, whether in the form of task lists, portals for access to completion, or interactive query documentation across the entire episode of care. The Level 3 EDMS system workflow will allow the clinicians to complete documentation within one single point of access for the entire record rather than attempting to complete in more than one location as frequently occurs within EHR applications that are non-HIM workflow-centric. One symptom that a system is designed inadequately to support deficiency analysis within HIM workflow appears when the software routes open records in a serial fashion to a clinician for authentication or completion instead of using criteria-based routing. In addition, inadequately designed systems do not provide detailed reports and statistics on volumes of outstanding records or delinquent aging reports to help manage incomplete records.

It is important to note that at the point of patient discharge in an episode of care, all documentation components, regardless of whether they are completed and authenticated, should be transferred via COLD feed into the EDMS to provide a complete documentation set and a single point of access for completion by the clinician. In cases where documents are not released from a source system until final completion, the documents are fragmented, resulting in a medical record in an incomplete state for an undetermined period of time, with no ability to track the stage of completeness. The impact of this incomplete state is far-reaching on the HIM department's deficiency analysis, coding, reimbursement, and release of information procedures and should not occur in a best practice environment.

There are two parts to deficiency analysis:

⊙ Document completion

⊙ Electronic signature

Document completion is the part of deficiency identification that occurs when a component of documents such as a note, report, or result, is missing within the patient record. When reviewing the complete record online, as components are noted as missing, the EDMS workflow software must allow the flagging or identification of the missing component as part of the deficiency processing.

Electronic signature is the second component of deficiency analysis. When a patient record is missing a signature there are several ways to obtain it. In some facilities, documents are still manually printed, and clinicians are allowed to authenticate or edit the documents by hand. This procedure is not recommended because the electronic source document still retains its original content without the amended version being available for a set amount of time. Although scanning the document may eventually take place, the gap in time raises a potential concern for patient care treatment based on incorrect information present in the electronic version. Therefore, to optimize the use of the EDMS software, it is recommended that the HIM workflow include a process to support the use of online electronic signature authentication and editing with a bidirectional feed to the source system as well as retained in the EDMS.

Loose or Late Report Processing

In the paper or hybrid environments, the processing of loose documents arriving separately from the main portion of the medical record chart after patient discharge is a large problem. Within electronic record environments, this problem diminishes or is less recognizable due to the information flow. Whereas each individual report would need to be filed into a separate paper folder or file, with an EDMS system that allows for scanning of documents, the reports that are received need only be sorted into those documents that still need to be scanned into the system, greatly reducing the time spent on this function. This is a major change in workflow process, and staff allocated to this function can be reassigned to other duties pertaining to EDMS processing. See chapter 5 for further review of changing job roles in the EDMS environment.

The documents that are received late or loose from the rest of the chart still need identification numbers assigned to them to ensure that they will be scanned in the correct sequence and for the correct encounter. The workflow software within the EDMS can be utilized as a time saver to make this verification task automatic as long as the account number is listed on each document. When a quick review of the chronological visit history is not available or is cluttered with clinic appointment or cancelation listings, it becomes increasingly difficult to determine the correct environment into which a single report should be scanned if it is missing an account number, thus decreasing the likelihood of a loose report ending up in the correct electronic file.

Incomplete Record Processing Considerations

After the deficiency process is completed, the medical records enter into a completed stage or into an incomplete stage. The term *delinquent record* is used to represent those records that have aged into a certain state in which the absence of documentation or authentication is beyond the time frame viewed as acceptable by the facility. These time frames—the standards by which incomplete records are judged—and the actions taken in response to a record becoming delinquent vary from facility to facility. The individual policies and procedures are based on medical staff guidelines, bylaws, policies, and procedures, as well as accreditation standards and state and federal government regulations.

As a fulfillment of a medical record deficiency for missing information, electronic signature authentication (ESA) is used to electronically sign documents both while they are in the EHR point of care documentation process, and retrospectively within the EDMS. ESA allows facilities to permit clinical providers to authenticate documents remotely rather than requiring them to physically work on a stack of incomplete records and apply numerous signatures on reports that they have previously dictated.

While all facilities encourage documentation to be completed in a timely manner, close to the delivery of actual patient care, some facilities are more tolerant than others in accepting late documentation and authentication. In the paper record environment, late entries in documentation and signature were difficult to track—if a date was not recorded at the time of notation or signature, the external reviewer could not tell if the documentation was recently added or present at the time of care delivery. However, with the advent of the EHR, entries are automatically assigned dates and times as the record is created, revised, or electronically signed. This creates a much more obvious audit trail and the deficiencies in this documentation become more glaring, with an emphasis made on reducing the amount and use of verbal orders, typically accounting for the bulk of missing signatures within a facility. In the most advanced facilities and innovative systems, the capture of this missing data is beginning to be addressed during the active patient care part of the encounter as a component of the clinical documentation improvement initiative, rather than addressing the capture of missing data as retrospective deficiency analysis and completion post discharge.

 The EDMS workflow software is built to monitor these documentation deficiencies, keep statistics on such occurrences, notify providers of issues, produce reports, lists, alerts, and reminders to clinicians, and otherwise ensure that the tracking of incomplete and delinquent records can be reported and reviewed closely for problem trends. This monitoring is often embedded and used in combination with deficiency processing notifications.

⊙ Best Practices and Innovation Takeaways

The MPI represents the point of entry and control of the patient's medical record into the healthcare system. The following checklist of questions can ensure that policies, procedures, and adequate audit control are implemented with the HIM department to address data and document integrity within the EHR or EDMS:

- ☑ Is there a daily duplicate medical record number and account number validity checking process in place? How are other functional areas, outside of the HIM department, notified of the duplication? How are the records merged in both a paper and electronic environment?

- ☑ Is there a daily chart reconciliation process in place for both collecting discharged paper records and reconciling electronic inputs and outputs into the document management system and overall EHR?

- ☑ Does the prepping and scanning process include checks for various documentation integrity issues such as missing reports, blurred images, and mislabeled documents?

- ☑ Does the MPI contain the correct number of entries, in the right sequence so that it has episode-of-care integrity within its account numbers?

- ☑ Are series and recurring patient registrations handled properly to avoid zero charge cases being present in the MPI?

- ☑ Does the deficiency analysis process occur before the function of coding and abstracting to assure records are not routed to a coder before the records are ready to be reviewed?

Ensuring that there are adequate controls in place to encourage data and document integrity are vital to an effective and efficient workflow.

REFERENCE

WebFinance, Inc. 2014. Workflow. http://www.businessdictionary.com/definition/workflow.html

Chapter 3

Advanced Health Information Management for EHR and EDMS Workflow

This chapter continues to review core workflow functions and processes within the health information management (HIM) department, with an emphasis on those that are more complex in nature. As such, these functions are even more dependent on the ability to view, manage, and print an accurately formatted medical record by specific page or section or in its entirety. These functions also typically utilize specific software applications to support the workflow processes:

⊙ Within the electronic health record (EHR) system itself,

⊙ Within the electronic document management system (EDMS) being used for the legal health record (LHR), or

⊙ Within a standalone other software system.

In each case, there is integration between these applications, the source system(s) from which the documentation in the medical record is created, and other legacy systems that may feed into the EHR, including other software applications and databases.

⊙ Coding, Grouping, and Data Abstracting Considerations

The heart of the HIM department may be viewed as its coding, grouping, and data abstracting functions since, during these functions, the true content of the documents within the medical record are most thoroughly reviewed and captured for statistical, epidemiological, and billing functions. This section describes the typical workflow of these functions as they transition into an electronic environment.

Coding and Grouping

The coding function encompasses review of the complete medical record and the subsequent assignment of appropriate alphanumeric codes based on various classification systems such as the International Classification of Diseases,10th Revision, Clinical Modification (ICD-10-CM) or Current Procedural Terminology (CPT) codes. An encoding system is typically used as a software assist tool to determine the correct formatting on the numeric code, based on clinical and demographic data supplied to the encoder software, either by a human coder or electronically through interfaced data systems. The grouping software, separate yet dependent on the encoder software, takes the output of coded data from the encoder and uses it to calculate expected reimbursement or potential compliance edits.

Specialized encoder and grouping software is used to supplement the coding process and this software integrates with the EDMS, EHR, and the overall health information system (HIS). This software may be integrated with the EDMS workflow software to ensure that demographic and account charge data is fully available within the application to support efficient review and coding processes. Work queue routings within the EDMS are essential to the coding function, since the goal is to have the coder touch the record a single time, as opposed to having to retrieve and review the episode more than once. These routings group a subset of electronic records together based on account number, service date, and service category. The routings are displayed in a work list that can automatically route the encounters in a prescribed order based on certain criteria or allow staff to pick an encounter and process it depending on the policies of the organization.

The coding function in a Level 3 EDMS environment has a distinct operational advantage over other settings that are not optimizing the use of EDMS workflow software and therefore have documents stored in different repositories or source systems. These efficiencies within the EDMS are created due to work queue routing and the availability of the complete record in a single electronic folder using a just-in-time methodology, which helps avoid redundant handling of the medical record by the various users.

There is often a misperception of the coding process in the industry. Individuals mistakenly believe that reviewing a subset or abstract of the medical record is sufficient and will result in complete coding of the record. Although there are certain documents that routinely contain information relative to coding along with other, less frequently used documents, the entire medical record must be available to the coders for review to produce the most accurate and compliant assignment of codes. In circumstances where the EDMS is not utilized as the legal health record and in situations where the electronic hybrid record exists but documentation is fragmented and stored in different source systems, there may be a tendency for coding staff to avoid taking the time to search out different documents for review, thus missing key information that changes, adds, or deletes a code.

The coding process is under continued severe scrutiny for compliance and extreme pressure for productivity improvement within facilities. This scrutiny has been heightened because of the anticipated long-term decrease in productivity relative to the adoption of ICD-10-CM and ICD-10-PCS. These pressures add to the propensity for bypassing reviews of documents that may be difficult to access or the acceptance of less than complete documentation, as in the case of late reports like discharge summaries, in order to be done with a single encounter review.

When planning the changes in workflow process for the coding area, setting up different categories, queues, work streams, or buckets—all are synonymous terms—is an essential step in preparing for the change in process. In the paper environment, stacks of charts would be assigned to various coders, most typically by discharge date. Backlogs readily occurred and tracking discharged not final billed (DNFB) days outstanding was challenging. With the advent of automation in the various health information systems and within the EDMS, HIM managers have the ability to use work queues to route the completed electronic records to the coding staff based on certain criteria such as highest dollars outstanding, or all of a certain clinic's discharges by date.

The best practice of ensuring coders do not code records until the process of deficiency analysis and completion of the record occurs has become a frequently ignored work routing practice with the adoption of the EHR. Based on personal surveys conducted by the author in the course of various facility interactions, approximately 40 percent of medical records must be returned for additional documentation in cases where work routing is not set up to perform analysis prior to coding, which results in the record being reviewed and handled more than once.

To correct this situation, there must be basic guidelines established in the facility of what is acceptable minimum content for coding. For example, are coders allowed to code with or without a discharge summary? Are coders allowed to code with or without a pathology report?

In addition, the routing queue should be set up to forward to the coding group after a specific number of days based on those guidelines. In this way, coders handle the record only a single time. Routing by determining queue categories is one of the most powerful tools in an EDMS. Setting up the appropriate routing queues within EDMS workflow can significantly improve productivity.

The determination of basic default queue sequencing takes place before the individual queues are determined. Typically, a common default queue will be set using first the oldest discharge date, and then the highest dollar amount within discharge date. This basic setting helps to route the individual encounters, one full record at a time, to the coders to ensure the lowest possible DNFB level for a facility.

Samples of coding-related queue categories with accompanying brief descriptions and benefits of such queues which should be developed when setting up the EDMS workflow include:

⊙ **Routing by patient type or work type.** Coders often specialize by patient type, which includes inpatients, diagnostic outpatients, observation or day surgery, emergency, series or recurring, clinic, and other types of services or visits. Routing by category allows similar records that require similar coding processing to be worked upon in sequence. This also provides the coder the ability to code from multi-facilities with same patient types when working in a remote multi-facility environment and maintain excellent productivity due to routing of these similar records.

⊙ **Routing by holding category.** As records are analyzed for deficiencies, they may need to be rerouted into a specific hold category. This category might be, for example, all encounters awaiting operative reports. When it is time to review and audit any queues as they age within the system, looking at like groups of charts helps the management of the process.

⊙ **Routing by review reason.** There may be specialty records that require additional reviews by an auditor, a manager, or another coder, such as a queue of records that are part of a normal internal audit or compliance program. For example, all records that contain a code for a complication due to a device may need to be routed to the internal risk manager prior to finalizing the coders. An EDMS allows the functionality to group such records, and route and manage the completion of those reviews based on calendar dates.

⊙ **Routing by financial class or payor.** Different coding rule variations or internal procedures might be set by financial class or payor. Creating an additional routing for workflow can assist with the management of cases in these areas.

⊙ **Routing by problem category.** The impact of data and document integrity errors are often felt most intensely in the coding area due to problems caused by MPI. If there is a duplicate account number, incorrect document on the encounter, erroneous discharge date, mistaken physician name on a report, wrong patient status as an observation instead of an inpatient, and so on, the coder will have difficulty moving forward. Being able to route and hold records into a problem category allows these issues to be categorized and managed within the EDMS workflow functions.

⊙ **Routing by facility.** Priority routing in a multi-facility environment can be difficult for many systems to handle due to confidentiality restrictions or separate technical server set-up. Remote coders are often trained to work on several facilities at a time. Coding vendors who provide this service in an outsourced fashion also may need to access encounters across facilities to track historical conditions and retrieve greater detail in, for example, oncology cases. The EDMS workflow layer allows complicated routing variation in facilities to be set up to accommodate differences in workflow, whether in a centralized or decentralized working environment.

Natural Language Processing—Computer Assisted Coding

Natural Language Processing (NLP), which is the use of automated tools to identify certain work patterns for various purposes, is advancing to the point where document identification, based on capturing narrative words or identification fields within a document, can be machine read and translated with a sufficient degree of accuracy to create the indexed identifier for document type capture within the EDMS. When used to assist with the process of coding, this technology is referred to as Computer Assisted Coding (CAC). In this way, large batches of electronic records, as opposed to scanned images, can be organized within a computer-assisted coding application and mimic the functionality of an EDMS as it pertains to creating an electronic record consisting of report-formatted templates captured in a static view, intermingled with scanned images of documents to create the full legal health record.

Many workflow efficiencies can be provided to the coding team through use of NLP and CAC technologies whether used in an environment devoid of EDMS technology or one that is utilizing a Level 1, 2, or 3 EDMS model. It is through the efficiencies of working with a complete document inventory during coding that many of the productivity gains of using NLP and CAC are recognized by an organization. Advanced processes such as the automatic coding, processing, queuing, availability, assignment, rerouting, and classifying coding cases that meet certain clinical, timing, or charge criteria may also be utilized in the coding process as a result of deploying NLP and CAC technologies.

When a Level 3 EDMS is in place, the feeds being integrated into the EDMS from the EHR can be dual-routed to the CAC application, thus avoiding a duplication of effort. This also provides for synchronization of results since they are available into the CAC software and the EDMS software simultaneously. The value perception of CAC software is higher in an environment not using a Level 3 EDMS since the CAC system can serve as a full document repository to help coders access the complete record as they had no other working solution. However, the efficiency gained in an HIM department for its staff is optimal when there is both a fully functioning EDMS utilizing all workflow functionality and a CAC system based upon solid principles of documentation and data integrity.

Data Abstracting

Abstracting of cases is typically performed by the coding staff during the coding process, but occasionally is performed as a completely separate task, after the coding process has taken place. *Abstracting* is the process of reviewing, editing, and otherwise ensuring certain data is collected on the patient relative to a specific encounter. Abstract summaries, which are a subset of all of the data in the medical record, are used to create the required indices that are used in hospitals to track diagnoses, procedures, mortality, physician activity level, and for other purposes.

Coding historically has been an epidemiological process, and indices were, and still are, used for statistical analysis of diagnosis and procedural trends and volume measurement. It is only within the past 30 years in the United States of America that coding information was used as part of the reimbursement process when prospective payment systems were introduced in the early 1980s. Abstracting data became a way to take the most critical parts of the patient record, using a combination of codes and other data to capture a brief summary for that patient.

The EDMS typically provides a vehicle to review the complete record from a single point of access while reading the story of the patient and ensuring all collected data is valid. Some of these systems are a part of the encoder and grouper suite of products; other times, the systems are embedded within the EDMS workflow functionality itself, and still other times the abstract summary is part of the health information system. Commingling information from previous episodes of care with an existing episode of care can be extremely problematic during coding and abstracting. For example, suppose that a problem list contains a diagnosis or medication that was present during a previous episode of care but has since been resolved. If the electronic documentation is not clear about the current status of the disease or drug, this information may be inadvertently coded and abstracted. As a result, a patient's insurance coverage and benefits (medical necessity conditions), legal custody determinations (presence of medication), driving status (diagnoses such as epilepsy), and even retention of a job may be negatively affected.

⊙ Clinical Documentation Improvement

Clinical documentation improvement (CDI) is the process of educating clinicians to document in the language of coding as opposed to the language of medicine. Prior to the advent of prospective payment systems and tying of codes to reimbursement, physician documentation quality was not used for coding detail in the same way it is today, since coding was purely epidemiological in nature. Today, there is a very close relationship between clinician (nurse, physician, and therapist, to name a few) and the health information management coder, because they depend on each other. The clinicians provide the content of the documentation via narrative words, and the coders translate the words into the coded numbers that are used for billing and statistics.

Clinical documentation improvement takes place both concurrently during the active episode of patient care as well as retrospectively after discharge and depends on the two groups to come together to tell the story of the patient. What are they being treated for, and what is being done for them to help them improve? Essentially, answering these questions, and documenting *why* something was ordered or done is at the core of a CDI program. The EHR may provide clues to be able to judge whether the documentation can support the diagnoses and explain any treatments provided to the patient, but the EHR's ever-changing dynamic and template-driven nature make it less than ideal as a platform for CDI. Ideally, the static nature of the Level 3 EDMS serves as a better viewing vehicle for retrospective coding and CDI purposes.

Regardless of whether an organization uses an EHR, an EDMS, or both systems, clinical documentation improvements can be introduced into the electronic medical record. For example a document that might include anatomical screening diagrams used upon registration into the facility may help to identify whether a condition was present on admission by allowing the clinician to document something as simple as a decubitus ulcer that is viewed on the skin of the patient during an initial exam. Drop-down menus and templates may aid physicians in selecting the right diagnosis or procedural documentation prior to sending the record to coding. Overall, clinical documentation and coding will become more successful as greater assistance is provided to clinicians to keep them current on documentation principles and easier querying processes, which serve as the primary communication tools between coders and physicians, are implemented.

⊙ Release of Information and Privacy Considerations

Releasing information is the workflow function most identified with privacy and security concerns within the EHR and may be considered the most time-consuming workflow component in the HIM department as the process needs to be done in multiple stages. Tasks such as obtaining patient consent, accumulating or gathering past records, and duplicating and distributing the record copies to requestors is labor intensive. People performing this workflow require a higher degree of specialization and training to properly process medical record query requests. Some facilities require a minimum of an RHIT or RHIA certification, or paralegal experience. Familiarity with state and national privacy guidelines, understanding all the locations for historical and present record storage, and the ability to work directly with the public—patients, as well as clinicians in a diplomatic way—are just part of the requirements. In a number of facilities, these individuals will also have to apply charging and collections rules and procedures due to the billable nature of health record requests.

These requests for release of information are often received years after the actual patient care episode, and thus stability and data integrity issues once again become critical on a long-term basis and cannot be supported by the dynamic, changing nature of a template-driven EHR. To fully support the legal health record, the stable nature of the EDMS is critical to a solid release of information process that protects patient privacy as well as the right to access information relative to a specific care encounter.

Release of Information

The release of information (ROI) function of the HIM department can potentially be one of the least understood workflow processes due to its complexity and voluminous state and federal regulations that influence this area. However, the EDMS function has a significant impact in supporting workflow for the ROI functions and can bring many workflow benefits to a facility.

The basic ROI function consists of a request or authorization from an individual or entity who wants to review a medical record or receive copies of that record. The request or authorization is followed by a response (also called a release) process on behalf of the provider that would then cause the facility to:

- Deny the request;
- Ask for clarification or a more specific authorization on the request; or
- Release the information requested either by paper, electronic or other media. In legal situations, the standards for subpoena and court order release primarily require a printed copy of a medical record from a single episode of care.

In certain circumstances there is also a monetary fee that may be charged for these services of releasing a copy of a record to a requestor. Charging a fee is dictated by specific state regulations that often have a set processing fee, a per-page fee, and mailing and supply costs that can be reimbursed to the copying organization. Since the physical paper- or software-based record is the property of the care organization and is their business evidentiary record, the patient does not own the original record. However, the patient has a right to review and access the content contained within that record and has a right to a copy of that record. Therefore, there is always a balancing act between the requesting and the releasing process for healthcare facilities to the requesting party. Typically there is no charge for continuity of care release of information between one provider and another provider.

To understand release of information principles, it is important to review, in more depth, the concept of the legal health record (LHR) that was introduced in chapter 1. In the release of information workflow, how the LHR definition is created will impact the workflow in the ROI process itself. The LHR can be described in more detail relative to ROI by stating:

> The legal health record (LHR) is defined as the subset of all patient-specific data created or accumulated by a healthcare provider that constitutes the organization's official business record, and is typically used when responding to formal requests for information for legal and legally permissible purposes. (Servais 2008)

To keep an LHR up to date requires continuous maintenance so that when any new form, documentation tasks, or other element of the medical record changes or is added to the facility, the LHR definition must also be updated.

There are many factors influencing the effectiveness of the release of information process, but none has as significant an impact as the use of an EDMS to provide a single platform and location from which to release any information from the official LHR. The easier the review and release process is, the more improved productivity is in doing the release, and the greatest risk mitigation occurs due to the ease of review of the entire record from a single unified location. It is in this way that there is little doubt as to the location of disparate records, since they are combined into a single processing and storage section within an EDMS.

Figure 3.1 is a checklist that can be used to identify some of the more important requirements in an EDMS in order to support ROI functions in an electronic record environment.

Figure 3.1   EDMS requirements checklist

☑ All documents can be accounted for and the record closed as complete within a specified time period post patient discharge.

☑ Single or multiple groups of documents within the electronic medical record can be viewed by or released to the requestor.

☑ An authorization for ROI can be visible at the episode-specific level affiliated with a specific encounter number.

☑ Global or universal authorizations can be filed at the enterprise (medical record number) level vs. individual episode of care.

☑ Documents can be reviewed through a portal, exported to a CD/DVD, or printed as a formatted output series of documents.

☑ Billing and collections process can be supported by the EDMS or accommodation made to integrate with the appropriate financial systems.

☑ A log of all requests and accounting of disclosures is kept as an audit trail and can be referenced as needed.

☑ External documents, which are either created digitally or scanned from paper into a system, can be integrated in a correspondence section of the electronic medical record within the EDMS.

Another driving factor to utilizing the EDMS as the legal health record to increase efficiency in the release of information process is as follows:

> Centers for Medicare and Medicaid Services (CMS) and the Office of the National Coordinator for Health IT (ONC) in August 2013 released the final rules and requirements for the stage 2 meaningful use EHR Incentive Program. Stage 1 required providers to give patients an electronic copy of their health information within three business days. In stage 2, this measure was modified to require that providers give patients the ability to *view online, download, and transmit their health information within 36 hours of discharge from the hospital*. The change increased the difficulty for HIM professionals working to release medical records. (Rollins 2013)

The rapid ability to gather and assemble all records—paper, electronic, or hybrid—and make the materials available for release electronically will be a challenge for hospitals that do not have a functional Level 3 EDMS in place to perform the ROI workflow process and provide full access to the LHR through the system. The processing time needed to review authorizations for validity and gather information in an EHR environment can be extremely time consuming. An external portal or a staffed internal viewing area will need to be made available seven days per week, creating some staffing and logistics concerns for departments who are located remotely from the care facility and might not be staffed in the ROI function seven days per week. And, those facilities still utilizing external contract or outsource services will need to determine to how to make those records available seven days per week.

Privacy

The Office for Civil Rights enforces the Health Insurance Portability and Accountability Act (HIPAA) Privacy Rule, which protects the privacy of individually identifiable health information (PHI); the HIPAA Security Rule, which sets national standards for the security of electronic protected health information; and the confidentiality provisions of the Patient Safety Rule, which protect identifiable information being used to analyze patient safety events and improve patient safety (HHS 2014). The HIM department is typically responsible for the functions of release of information and privacy in most healthcare organizations. This ombudsman, protector, and service role surrounding maintenance of the electronic record is a historical carry-over from the concept referred to as legal guardian or custodian of the record.

> The custodian of an electronic health record (EHR) has the same concerns as the custodian of a paper health record. The custodian of the legal health record is the health information manager in collaboration with information technology personnel. HIM professionals oversee the operational functions related to collecting, protecting, and archiving the legal health record, while information technology (staff) manages the technical infrastructure of the electronic health record. (AHIMA 2005)

Today, this accountability, along with other responsibilities of the HIM manager, is encompassed in the concept of health information governance, and the Level 3 EDMS provides a tool with which to operationalize and support this concept.

Privacy, at an operational level, means the custodian of the records must confirm that there are policies and procedures in place to guarantee that access to medical record content—specifically PHI—is held confidential. These policies and procedures can be as simple as ensuring that patient names are not used in physician office sign-in logs or displayed on a whiteboard at a nursing unit in a hospital. At a more complex level, these policies and procedures require prudent visible access and print controls throughout the EHR and EDMS. The technology used to create visible access and implement print controls must support an environment that allows limited access to PHI on a need-to-know basis within the guidelines of the laws governing release of information.

The need-to-know principle of privacy in healthcare applies to clinical staff (that is, physicians, nurses, ancillary personnel) as well as administrative staff in provider facilities. These individuals have a right to access information only if:

⊙ They are identified by role within the EHR, EDMS, or LHR as a member of the healthcare team that is currently treating the patient and has a need to access the medical record of that patient

⊙ They have a current authorization from the patient to access the patient's PHI

⊙ They have power of attorney or are a legal guardian for another individual

⊙ They need access to the content of the record to perform their job or role function, whether in a provider, consultant, auditor, or other staff function

The Level 3 EDMS supports the privacy concept through the workflow application in its software and hierarchical levels of access, and audit tracking can be provided across the medical record as a single entity. If the record were subdivided and kept as individual components within different functional applications, it would be difficult to provide protection or track numerous access audit logs. There are multiple facilities that may be using software that violates this concept of need-to-know PHI access, and thus are in overall violation of the rights that HIPAA attempts to protect. A violation of the HIPAA controls might occur when there is an overdependence on random retrospective access audit trails as the only indicator of PHI access violation instead of controlling the access actively. To prevent this violation of HIPAA controls, ensure access is only on a need-to-know basis for caregivers that are actively treating the patient during as episode of care and listed as providers on their record or unit of service.

Consider these specific situations relative to access to patient medical records that can be viewed as risk-prone and lacking appropriate consideration and controls for patient privacy and confidentiality if allowed within an EHR system:

⊙ Access to patient medical record data by nurses who may be working on a different nursing unit than the patient, but still have the ability to retrieve the online record of a patient and review it

⊙ Access to patient data on a nursing unit after the patient has been discharged

- Access to patient medical record data by physicians who are not active physicians of care on the case
- Access to past patient medical history data by physicians who have not seen the patient, do not have plans to see the patient, and have no patient authorization
- Access by family members or friends to patient medical record data without consent from the patient

Healthcare facilities may rationalize the need to provide open access to patient records under the guidance that there is no authorization or consent form needed for clinical care. However, since there can be no care provided unless there is an established relationship with the patient, this access is not legitimate. If a provider is actively involved in care, he or she can be established as a physician of record, and then can gain access to a patient's record in an urgent situation.

Another rationalization used to justify open access to clinicians who are not listed as a physician of record is the need to access information in an emergent situation where there may be no time to record a change in physician of record. In these cases, a best practice recommendation is to deploy a "break the glass" approach in which an individual may access a record, even if not listed as a clinician of record, by selecting an emergency access or bypass feature within the system. These cases are then automatically flagged for appropriate audit access review and validated, avoiding the random access audit and providing the ability to collect statistics around access activity levels.

In addition to access rights, printing rights often become a controversial topic in facilities. One facility may choose to provide printed access only through a central release of information function. Another facility may provide unlimited printing access to anyone who has the rights to review information as long as an audit trail tracks the printing performed. The practical, but real issue, of cost of printing copies—the paper and ink, as well as the equipment and its support—often influences the printing policies in place at a facility. The medical record in an electronic environment typically has many more pages of information printed than the older version paper records, adding to the cost of this printing.

The real issue of risk in an EHR or EDMS that allows decentralized printed copies is that the paper copies may be utilized in patient care instead of the practitioner viewing the online version. Some facilities provide a different color or marked type of paper in printers to identify that a printed record is not the original. Other facilities have a built-in workflow feature that identifies any printed copies as a duplicate next to the print information.

If the electronic online version is the legal health record, and all edits, modification, and final versions of documents are online, a person who uses the paper copy potentially can be working from erroneous information. Sites that generate portions of the medical record electronically but permanently archive their LHR in paper run an additional risk of printing an incorrect or duplicate version of the record. It is not unusual to observe HIM staff sorting out a hard copy record received from a nursing unit upon discharge and disposing of large number of pages of duplicate reports generated as a result of overzealous printing. Facilities utilize guidelines regarding this printing and disposal of extra documents as part of the policies that guide their LHR to mitigate this liability risk.

 The electronic document management system ROI workflow functionality helps to control access to retrospective medical record review through centralized organization of the documents. It is in this manner that protected health information within the legal health record can be protected as an episodic entity of care in full. All of the functionality necessary to manage the full document access and trails and providing the correct level of documentation around disclosures can be accomplished in the EDMS solution when utilized as the legal health record.

⊙ Chart Management

This section discusses the movement of the medical record available to providers and staff of a healthcare facility as an operational business record, exclusive of the process of externally releasing information. There exists a misperception in the industry that there is no need to provide chart-tracking functionality if permanent *paper* files are not being generated. Just as release of information functions in an electronic record must protect privacy, chart-management functions help to provide an audit trail identifying who has reviewed a record and for what purpose. As a facility is evolving from a paper to a hybrid and eventual electronic environment, patient chart management encompasses a variety of functions, including but not limited to the following tasks:

- ⊙ Paper and electronic file requests
- ⊙ Paper and electronic file retrieval
- ⊙ Paper and electronic file tracking
- ⊙ Paper and electronic file auditing
- ⊙ Archive and retention processes
- ⊙ Purge processes
- ⊙ Destruction processes

The paper and electronic file tasks are described in detail in the following sections. See chapter 7 for a more detailed discussion on medical record archive, retention, purge, and destruction issues.

Paper and Electronic File Requests

Paper and electronic file requests are similar in both the paper and the electronic environments, but efficiency is greatly improved with the use of workflow software applications within the EDMS. Medical records are reviewed extensively after patient care is complete. Reasons for this review may include quality of care, morbidity or mortality review, incident review, random or focused audits, staff or employee monitoring or investigations, research studies, documentation reviews, charge audits, or a multitude of other reasons. Data are often collected and extracted or abstracted from the medical record and entered into another database or registry.

Requests routinely are received in either a paper or electronic environment in the following ways:

- Receipt of a list via in person delivery, fax, or e-mail
- Online requests through specific software designed for this purpose
- Telephone and verbal requests

Paper and Electronic File Retrieval

In the paper environment or in a hybrid environment, a physical search must be completed to locate and retrieve the requested records by reviewing the master patient index to locate the specific episode of care being requested. This process is similar to what must be done in the release of information workflow to locate a specific episode of care.

When processing medical records electronically within an EDMS, there is a degree of indexing that is done on both the specific documents and other data elements. Some data elements are indexed automatically, while other data elements are indexed manually. The benefit of case indexing is the ability to drill down to retrieve a specific portion of a record or to filter the record using specific criteria during selection.

For example, suppose that a reviewer wanted to retrieve records of female patients within a certain visit date range who had a diagnosis of diabetes. If the encounter was specifically indexed to the demographics (that is, patient gender) and coded data (in this example, diabetes) for each episode of care (the discharge date range in this example), this criteria could be utilized to queue and retrieve an exact match to requestor criteria without performing a separate search to identify matching patients for audits or other information. These discrete data elements that are linked to each specific account provide the advanced functionality inherent in a Level 3 EDMS system workflow for chart management.

In the EDMS environment, the requestor is presented with the index of patient accounts within the MPI so that he or she can select and request the appropriate episode(s) of care if the encounter number or medical record numbers are already known to the requestor, creating an electronic queue of medical records. The requested records can automatically become available for review upon request if the records are all electronic in nature, or the request can go through a manual screening to verify the legitimacy of the request.

Housing the records within the EDMS allows the entire record to be available as a unit and from a single source to the requestor, instead of attempting to retrieve various portions of documentation, notes, and results and assemble them from various source systems often housed together loosely in an EHR. The action of creating the request sparks simultaneous queuing of records to create an audit trail for disclosure tracking. Standing requests can be kept and accessed in the future using previously created criteria for retrieval, significantly reducing the time spent on this step in the request and retrieval process due to the EDMS workflow.

Setting controls to prevent reviewers from printing or altering the record content are put into place to further verify the integrity of the record through a variety of means, including utilizing an EDMS solution since the EDMS solution typically has a built-in control that limits the ability of individuals to provide changes to a set document image once it is finalized. Other controls include visible documentation when any report is signed or amended, displaying the user's name, changes, and date of the change.

Paper and Electronic File Tracking

In cases where paper-based records are used, these medical records will need to be retrieved and presented to the reviewer. Additional tools are used in these environments such as chart tracking systems and outguides for file management controls. Chart tracking systems allow the technician retrieving the nonelectronic media to track the movement of the record by using bar coding or keyed data entry to identify the location of the current record. For example, a paper record may first exist in the permanent file within the HIM department. If a requestor from a nursing unit is reviewing the record for an audit, the paper record's location may be updated on a certain date to show it is "in the audit workroom on 2 N." When the record is returned to the original location, the record is refiled where it was retrieved, and the tracking location is updated to show the audit trail back to the permanent file.

Chart management theory is important to understand since there is a relationship between the EDMS and the paper records in a hybrid system: both must be used together to obtain the complete record from a chart tracking perspective. Another aspect of chart management that is important to relate to EDMS is the correlating electronic movement of the record as part of disclosure tracking. Just as someone who looked at a chart tracking application to see where the medical record was moved and for what purpose as the chart tracking was updated, the movement of the record in terms of who requested and reviewed it in various queues becomes the disclosure accounting and audit trail in the EDMS workflow.

Outguides are used to identify physical chart removal from a file system as a control in the paper world, and these are replaced in the electronic environment with work lists that show the records that have been checked out electronically and identify the reviewer, thus creating an audit trail. There are two types of outguides used in a paper filing system. The first is the file outguide, which is used as a temporary placeholder in a filing system so that the physical medical record is returned to the proper location. The other outguide tool is a three-ply outguide slip. The slip is marked to indicate the location to which the record is being moved. The first slip is attached to the medical record. The second slip is placed in the file outguide to identify which record was removed in lieu of the placeholder guide. The third slip is used as file control to guarantee records are returned after a specified number of days. The need for either of these systems and tools completely disappears with the use of an EDMS.

Paper and Electronic File Auditing

Where paper records still exist, the need for monitoring and auditing these records will also still exist. Routing audits that check for potentially misfiled records is one type of common audit. Using color-coded folders and labels assists with effective audits, along with labeling that includes the year of the last encounter. When the EDMS is adopted for use as the LHR as within a Level 3 EDMS, the need to audit paper files completely disappears because paper files on shelves are no longer retained long term, and the EDMS becomes the legal health record until the electronic file is purged. If an organization does not utilize the EDMS as the LHR, this audit function and the need to maintain a paper record may still exist for use by the organization as the LHR. This data integrity audit is replaced in the EDMS by the electronic reconciliation process described in the Missing Records section of this chapter, to ensure that all content of the medical record is received and complete.

⊙ Best Practices and Innovation Takeaways

Use the following checklist of best practices software functionality when evaluating an electronic health record system or electronic document management system vendor:

- ☑ Provides bidirectional interfaces between the encoder and grouper and the main health information system through abstracted and billed data.

- ☑ Provides work routing or queuing that accommodates multiple levels of filters.

- ☑ Provides linkages between analysis, deficiency management, transcription, and coding functionality to promote a complete and authenticated record.

- ☑ Provides a link between the clinical documentation software and encoder to support improved documentation, electronic routing of queries to physicians, and incorporating addenda in the electronic health record in a compliant manner.

- ☑ Provides full release of information management functionality, including tracking receipt of requests, gathering electronic medical records from all facilities, and processing those files, the billing and collections associated with the release, and the actual distribution of the copies of the records.

- ☑ Provides full chart management functionality to verify the identification or location of the source of the release, completeness of the documents being released, and destination for the release or review are available in the ROI software.

- ☑ Utilizes CAC and NLP technologies in addition to a fully functioning Level 3 EDMS and ensure access to documentation is synchronized between both software applications.

In summary, electronic document management systems that provide HIM workflow applications represent a powerful set of innovative tools that can be used as the legal health record. These complex tools within the EDMS help to provide a new level of efficiency, make managing the health record easier, and simplify request and retrieval processes. Coding, grouping, abstracting, clinical documentation improvement, release of information, and chart management workflow within the EDMS provides an effective solution in migrating from the paper to the hybrid and eventually a fully electronic environment that supports the legal health record within the EDMS and the EHR.

REFERENCES

AHIMA e-HIM Work Group on Defining the Legal Health Record. 2005 (October). The legal process and electronic health records. *Journal of AHIMA* 76(9):96A–D.

Department of Health and Human Services. 2014. Health Information Privacy. http://www.hhs.gov/ocr/privacy/

Rollins, G. 2013 (January). Road map to 2013: A guide through exciting but unfamiliar HIM territory and times. *Journal of AHIMA* 84(1):25.

Servais, C.E. 2008. *The Legal Health Record*. Chicago: AHIMA.

Chapter

4

The Human Component of Electronic Health Record Management in Healthcare

Effective change management of human resources is an essential element of any project involving large scale workflow and technology adoption, particularly in electronic health record management (EHRM). There is a tendency by some individuals or organizations in the healthcare industry to focus on the bells and whistles such as the technological components of an electronic health record (EHR) system instead of identifying aspects of workflow changes on the facility and their impact on the workforce. Software that helps to automate tedious and time-consuming tasks and improve the quality and data integrity of the medical record is indeed exciting. Implementation of an electronic document system (EDMS) as a vital component of the EHR involves significant process changes for the health information management (HIM) staff as well as clinicians and other users of the medical record. This chapter explores the human component of organizations that attempt either EHR or EDMS innovation.

⊙ Overview

Features and functions of software rapidly change, and facilities often undertake multiple product upgrades or purchase several new solutions in a single year, some of which overlap in functionality in certain areas as the products evolve. However, how well a facility ultimately performs in conjunction with their technical solution of choice has much to do with the human element, including the physical workspace and the culture of the purchasing organization. From the moment a decision is made to progress down the path of HIM workflow automation and provide for an electronic legal health record, the needs of the workforce must be considered throughout the selection process, planning, implementation, and post go-live activities.

The journey typically begins with a philosophical discussion as to how the workflow changes will be addressed and what the physical work environment will be like for the HIM team, because the environment will certainly look and feel different than the one that supports the paper or hybrid record version present in most facilities today.

This discussion then progresses to resources and space, identifying the workstations, equipment, and supplies that will be needed and deciding whether to utilize a centralized or a noncentralized approach in the use of the EDMS. As the changing job roles are identified, new job requirements and descriptions need to be written and potential changes in pay scales relative to new skills or educational mandates need to be addressed. Addressing these changes may be particularly challenging in environments that utilize unions, and the time needed to make these changes should not be underestimated. Refer to chapter 5 for a discussion of these changes in job roles that should be considered.

Simultaneous to these environmental changes taking place within the HIM department, the project leaders must address facility-wide key stakeholders and create a steering committee to help guide and monitor the success of the project. While this may seem like a relatively simple task, complex political cultures, internal authoritative hierarchy, and conflicting departmental or facility priorities may make this a significant challenge.

 Determining how best to involve the HIM staff, clinicians, and other departmental professionals in this project from the onset will help minimize any negative impact experienced as a result of large-scale system changes simply due to the extended buy-in to a project that involvement naturally brings.

While there are long-term needs for the work staff to address once the EDMS system is ready for implementation—such as training, the development of new policies and procedures, and so on—there are additional and more subtle dimensions to supporting the human elements of change that this chapter will explore so that the reader can optimize his or her environment for successful implementation and use of an EDMS in his or her own facility.

⊙ Changing Work Environments: The Physical Department

In a smaller facility or a physician's clinic, EDMS may be focused more upon the conversion of the documents from paper into images instead of on the actual workflow functions as was previously discussed in chapters 2 and 3. The changes in workflow are minimal, and paper documents simply *scanned* after completion, as opposed to being filed onto shelving units. Documents also may be directly imported from an electronic medical record (EMR) charting template or come from dictated reports stored within the clinical charting system. Guided by an individual organization's policies, these paper documents are either destroyed immediately upon scanning, or stored temporarily until a certain destruction date and time. The addition of a scanner may be the only physical change in the office.

However, when a hospital makes the decision to move along the automation continuum for electronic health information management (e-HIM™), the physical work environment, as well as the workflow, equipment, and supplies used in that environment, change in a significant way. Understanding those changes and how they impact the workforce is an important part of the planning process for implementing and using an EDMS. Architects, internal space and facility planning experts, and consultants are helpful if a larger redesign project is indicated. Consider the following factors in planning the conversion to an EDMS environment from a current paper or hybrid environment.

Physical Environment

The change to the physical environment within the HIM department begins with planning the physical workflow and department design with the goals of understanding the volume of records flowing through the system and planning out adequate desk and work space. Provide enough room to process the paper medical records received from the patient care units post discharge, since these paper records will still exist even in the most automated of settings. The volume of paper associated with these post-discharge records invariably decreases as more and more clinical documents originate from an electronic source system. The processing or staging area is the first area of change to consider when redesigning physical environments to accommodate an EDMS implementation and should be designed with adequate space for incoming medical records as the patients are discharged from the patient care areas or clinics.

As the medical records are collected or received in the immediate post-discharge time frame into the HIM department, they must be processed and temporarily stored. Open shelving that is divided into area by discharge date best houses these records. Utilizing temporary traveling folders for these collected records is a common practice that helps to separate the stacks of paper, which can be quite large. Storage shelves may also be needed to store routing forms, folders, separator pages, supplies, and any other additional materials associated with the prepping tasks. Special shelving and filing folders such as accordion hanging files or bin storage can be used for this type of temporary storage as well. Mobile shelving units previously used for long-term paper medical record storage can be repurposed for this type of storage, typically requiring far fewer units than previously used for indefinite long-term record retention. Repurposing and reconfiguring expensive shelving hardware to support this post-discharge temporary processing storage need can recycle existing items as well as save considerable expenditures for a facility.

Since records may be received into a central area in relatively large volumes, access to a dock with truck delivery and cart ramps must be considered if the physical location of the centralized work area is located at a considerable distance from the patient care areas. Access to a dock with truck delivery and cart ramps is particularly helpful if the processing area is a centralized one supporting multiple facilities. With a limit of no more than two driving hours separating the offsite processing center from the satellite facilities that are centralizing their operations, health information departments are able to optimize their processing schedules. The two-hour distance maximum limit recommendation serves to accommodate efficient and timely chart pick-up and delivery schedules, including urgent retrieval for patient care purposes in sites that do not have immediate scanning capabilities around the clock.

Security is essential to any area that houses records and record-processing activities, so identification badge entry to keypad security entry is recommended for access in and out of the building. Security cameras are recommended for truck docking areas, and mirrored reflectors should be in place for any file storage areas within the processing center where direct visibility doesn't exist while staff is working with protected health information documents such as the medical records.

Typically up to 90 processing days post discharge can be used as an estimate for storage needs in this temporary area as a best practice for staging of paper records prior to destruction once the record has been scanned. To calculate the linear inches needed, take the average number of inches in a day's discharge, multiply by 5 percent growth times 90 days (Stewart 2014). Include all outpatient and inpatient record volumes that need to be processed. Avoid using the highest and lowest shelves to speed processing and access time. Facilities typically conduct a quality audit prior to destroying the original paper records by examining a 10 percent sampling of the paper records against the electronic file to assure a 100 percent accuracy match. Any errors identified will cause the entire box or batch of records to be audited and all inconsistencies corrected before purging paper records.

Dividers to separate types of records, such as emergency department or day surgery charts, are helpful in larger operations. This practice of using dividers is not very different than a routine centralized paper-based processing area within an HIM department, except that the folders, if used, are not prepped with color coded labels, year bands, and other supplies typically seen and used in a paper environment. In some of the processing environments, the paper charts that await scanning and quality checks are actually stacked vertically, without separation of folders, and housed in stacks or in boxes by day. If multiple dates exist in a single shelving system, they are also separated and clearly delineated by a date divider to help locate records. Although 90 days does not seem like a lot of time, the temporary storage needs for these active records can be significant in a larger environment that processes hundreds or thousands of patients per day.

This processing area is used to perform reconciliation by comparing received records to discharge lists from the previous day to ensure all patient records have been successfully collected and transferred from the clinical area to the HIM processing area.

As the records from each discharge date are processed, that stage of processing can be checked off on a processing checklist. See figure 4.1 for a sample of a form that can be used to keep turnaround-time statistics for each of the key processing steps. This checklist, when used, has a designated label for each batch of records being processed on the shelves, and serves to notify anyone that may be accessing the area of the activity level of the discharged records. For example, staff performing

Figure 4.1   EDMS processing checklist

DISCHARGE DATE: _____

TOTAL INPATIENT MEDICAL RECORDS: _____

Reconciled Against Discharge List: Yes   No   Initials: _____

If No: List Missing Encounter Numbers: (Note date received if received late.)

DATE PREPPED: _____   TOTAL INCHES: _____
Initials: _____

DATE SCANNED/INDEXED: _____   TOTAL SIDES of PAGES: _____
Initials: _____

DATE QUALITY CHECKED: _____   DATE DESTROYED: _____
Initials: _____   Initials: _____

TOTAL OUTPATIENT MEDICAL RECORDS: _____

Reconciled Against Discharge List: Yes   No   Initials: _____

If No: List Missing Encounter Numbers: (Note date received if received late.)

functions like release of information may need this information to determine whether a record should be released if it has not yet gone through the deficiency analysis process as described in chapter 2.

After records are processed, they are commonly placed in a storage container or box labeled with the discharge date, type of record, and estimated destruction date. (Refer to chapter 7 for discussion of record retention issues.)

Workstations and Equipment

After the processing area is adequately planned, the next consideration should be the workstations and equipment. Some items that are already used in the facility may be repurposed; new purchases will need to be planned for others.

The technicians responsible for processing the record are the only personnel that must be physically located near the processing area. The technical process includes the prepping, scanning, indexing, quality control, and destruction processes being performed on the documents. All other functions within the HIM department that are dependent upon review of the medical record can be located remotely, because the record is completely electronic and accessible in multiple locations once this step is completed.

Planning adequate numbers of workstations once again depends on the volume of records to be processed and the time standards used for the processing. As a facility determines the correct number of workstations, they should be laid out with the following considerations:

- ⊙ All workstation locations should have room to accommodate double monitors for staff use.

- ⊙ All workstations should have space for appropriate individual scanners or high-speed, larger capacity scanners.

- ⊙ All workstations should have access to centrally located printers, copiers, and other equipment.

- ⊙ Processing areas should be located in quiet areas that do not experience interruptions from telephones, walk-in inquiries, or other distractions, because staff needs a high level of concentration to ensure data integrity during the processing.

- ⊙ Desk areas should be large enough to accommodate spreading out documents while processing a high volume of paper.

- ⊙ Workstations can ideally be shared up to three full shifts per day, seven days per week to minimize space footprint for workflow.

- ⊙ The ideal workstation height is five to six feet to incorporate some privacy between workstations.

- ⊙ Both desk lighting and overhead lighting are necessary elements to consider in workstation design.

- ⊙ Electrical needs can be considerable at each workstation and should include a minimum of eight outlets per workstation. Individual requirements should be evaluated by an electrician.

- ⊙ Access to high-speed and high-bandwidth telecommunications lines is essential to the success of an EDMS implementation. Consultation with information technology professionals familiar with the facility infrastructure, the vendor who is providing the software solution and external consultants is recommended.

- ⊙ Any redesign and new workflow provides the opportunity to physically modernize the area to make it attractive and provide a motivational environment in which to work. The switch from paper records or a hybrid environment to a fully automated workflow to HIM may provide a rare opportunity to update the department design. The personnel in HIM are primarily sedentary, so the need for sturdy, functional, and comfortable ergonomic chairs is essential to a healthy workforce. Consulting an architect for additional subject matter and design input is recommended.

⊙ Adequate restroom, break room, meeting or training room, and locker space is another essential aspect of the record processing area.

Some of the larger-sized equipment and the various supplies used within an EDMS environment are the same as those used in the paper process, while others are different. Understanding the differences between the equipment and supplies used in each processing environment is important to planning the budget and space of a redesigned physical environment. Adequate space must be planned at both the workstation level as well as within the central shared work areas where larger equipment such as a high-speed copy machine may be located. A more detailed discussion of technical requirements related to the EDMS can be found in chapter 9.

In the paper world, file folders with color-coded labels are a large expenditure to the HIM department. With an EDMS system, other than the files used in temporary storage during the initial processing, permanent file folders are no longer needed because the paper records are destroyed a short time after being scanned into the EDMS. Therefore, storage areas for empty folders, prongs and labels, and equipment designed to produce such labels also are no longer needed.

The scanning equipment required to convert plain paper to an electronic image, dual-sided paper to two images, photographs into an electronic image, colored paper into a readable image, and other specialty forms will need to be considered based on the mix of particular forms output in each facility. The speed of the scanning equipment needed will vary based on the volume of records. Individual scanners can be used for small amounts of paper to be processed, such as scanning loose and late reports into the EDMS. Larger scanners allow high-speed batch or bulk scanning, without requiring that each record be inserted separately. High-speed batch or bulk scanning can only be accomplished if records are properly identified with the appropriate demographic and form identification on the form itself or on a cover indexing document.

One of the greatest misconceptions about electronic records is that they no longer will need to be printed. Very often, either portions of or the entire EHR will need to be printed to review, transfer copies of the record, or provide a duplicate hard copy record for requestors in the release of information process.

Therefore, high-speed laser printers, capable of handling copious amounts of paper printing, will be necessary. As medical records are automated within the EHR, printing occurs more frequently, necessitating an adequate number of printers. The software components of the EHR that integrate electronically via computer output laser disk (COLD) into the EDMS also add to the increase in print volume. Also plan and allot space for high-speed fax servers that are capable of routing copies of the medical records and receiving input from other facilities. The use of faxing in healthcare is extremely prevalent, particularly for receiving and sending documents between physician office settings and hospitals and other care organizations. Faxing often occurs because of the high volume of requests for information; the need to receive various records, orders, and requests; and the lack of interoperability in systems between these facilities.

Rather than using only a printer, a high-speed copier should also be available to photocopy duplicates of a printed record, particularly to meet release of information requests. A best practice tip is to use paper within the copy machine or printer that is pre-marked with *duplicate* on the paper, designated with a colored strip, or printed directly onto colored paper to differentiate the non-original paper version of the medical record from an original source document. Since the legal health record (LHR) would be considered the online electronic version in an EHR environment, differentiating the LHR from the paper copies avoids confusion or use of the incorrect version of the document.

⊙ Centralized Compared to Decentralized Environments

Considering whether a department will be operating in a centralized or decentralized manner or in a combination thereof is an important consideration in planning the revised physical workspace and workflow in an EDMS environment. Larger work areas are needed in the centralized environment, since the workforces and the incoming volume of discharged medical records of several locations may merge. Note that this combining of workforces can save space in each facility respectively and provide added benefit from sharing equipment and resources, offering better economies of scale in managing the centralized configuration.

In a physically centralized environment, various functions of the department are physically located together, and perform the functions of the department as a team. For example, all scanning, release of information, analysis, or other functions for multiple facilities is handled by a single team in a single physical location. In a physically decentralized environment, there can be a single team that is located remotely, or there can be multiple teams, reporting to multiple areas of management. For example, a healthcare system may have three hospitals with each of them having their own HIM department manager, all of whom report to the same individual or different individuals. These departments may or may not be cross-trained to cover processing functions for the other facilities; further, they may or may not be guided by the same policies or even medical staff regulations.

Centralized management of the HIM functions refers to the single source management of certain functions. In decentralized print control, for instance, printing duplicate copies of the paper output of the medical record may take place in a number of different locations. Centralized print control is designed to manage the print functions from a single location. With the exception of some decentralized scanning input for pre-registration documentation and consent form receipt, supporting policy and procedure consistency and data integrity is considered best practice for centralized HIM management throughout the EDMS process. Economies of scale for training and staffing are also supported by a more centralized approach.

Centralized and decentralized physical locations may ultimately be determined by the availability of space or resources. Functions that benefit from physical centralization are typically those that share equipment or personnel. The cost of four staff members sharing a single printer is less expensive than each member having his or her own piece of equipment.

The volume of records being processed and the number of facilities involved is another consideration that will help a site decide if the centralized or the decentralized style is best for the site. If there are groups of physician clinics or multiple facilities within an integrated delivery network, combining functions and management in a central location may make more sense.

Various workflow functions have differing advantages and disadvantages when performed in a centralized or a decentralized environment. In some cases, combination models may exist that may best benefit the facility. Table 4.1 presents examples of advantages and disadvantages for the various elements of workflow within different processes within the HIM department.

As hospitals become more automated, the ability to remotely manage HIM work teams either centrally or disparately, away from the physical campus of the main patient care delivery areas, becomes a reality, thus creating virtual HIM campuses.

⊙ Stakeholders

In poker games, raising the stakes refers to increasing the bet, which, in turn, makes the hand at play increasingly important to the players at the tables. When considering stakeholders relative to an EDMS project, identifying the appropriate individuals certainly brings value to the project because the buy-in of these stakeholders is essential to the successful selection, purchase, implementation, and use of the EDMS in the healthcare facility.

The stakeholders for an EDMS project are those individuals that can be classified primarily in three categories:

- ⊙ Those who are subject matter experts or have knowledge about the project
- ⊙ Those who have control and authority over the project, such as those who assign or release resources, including funding
- ⊙ Those who directly or indirectly influence the success of the project

Subject matter experts consist primarily of the HIM departmental leadership because of their familiarity with the detailed workflow to support the management of the medical record, as well as their role as the official custodian of the legal health record. However, additional subject matter experts will be needed throughout the planning and life cycle of document management, such as ancillary leadership from any number of clinical departments who will be providing documentation *into* the medical record. Unless an external consultant, vendor, or other specialist

Table 4.1   Comparison of EDMS centralized vs. decentralized workflow environments for some key functions: benefits and disadvantages

FUNCTION	CENTRALIZED	DECENTRALIZED	COMBINATION
Document scanning	Consistent process; sharing of staff resources, equipment, and space.	Allows quicker entry (at point of care), but may not be a primary job focus so quality may suffer. Prepping may be difficult to perform.	Preregistration and consent documents can be pre-entered for multiple access and view.
Analysis	Specially trained staff can process records remotely, but under a centralized management infrastructure.	Dedicated individuals specializing in a certain unit's function can be assigned. May double as unit secretaries for concurrent completion activities.	Possibility that both functions can simultaneously exist to reduce record deficiencies, and provide for prompt processing.
Coding	Coders can easily assist each other in a central physical location. Communication, training, and quality checks are easier in this environment.	Recruitment and retention may benefit from a decentralized approach employing remote employees. Productivity often increases for remote workers.	The dual option or part onsite, part offsite has proven successful. If technical problems occur, having an on-site alternative is also helpful for the coding staff.
Release of information	Centralized access, particularly if physically near older paper files as well as electronic access, can speed productivity in this area. This model can help eliminate use of expensive outsource/contract labor for release of information.	As records become fully electronic, the options for remote worker support is a possibility. Access portals and "walk in" stations located near patient registration provide higher levels of customer-focused service.	Control for authorization, release consents, and printing provide higher levels of privacy, security, compliance and confidentiality for the patient.

who has worked with HIM workflow in an EHR and EDMS environment is used to help guide the facility through this change process, the EDMS or EHR project teams may suffer from a lack of practical knowledge as they begin an implementation.

Additional expertise from a technical point of view may also be provided by telecommunications, information technology, and physical plant maintenance staff concerning the electrical and design considerations for wiring, communications, and physical space redesign.

Those stakeholders who have control, authority and funding approval of the EDMS project are most likely the chief financial officer, chief executive officer, chief information officer, and chief medical officer. Subject matter experts must interact with these stakeholders to create awareness of the workflow requirements and help to educate this team of executives on the use of the EDMS as a vital component of the EHR.

There may be a gap in knowledge at the executive level about the differences between a Level 3 EDMS when compared to a scanning or imaging system and the need for advanced workflow functionality to support some of the requirements of the legal health record and ensure productivity standards are met within HIM processing. This knowledge gap is particularly serious if the team of executives had been thinking that the EHR without an EDMS would be able to meet the workflow needs. The subject matter experts must be sensitive to this relearning, because the evolution in thinking about the use of document management systems as a vital component is just emerging in the industry.

The final group of stakeholders is the influencing group. These are typically users of the medical record who have a personal, vested interest in the changes an EDMS may bring to their individual workflow and medical record review needs. Their primary contact with the medical record is typically as a user providing documentation into the EHR or as a reviewer who requests and utilizes the content of the medical record from a view context. They may have difficulty accepting or visualizing changes in an electronic environment because they may be comfortable with existing paper or hybrid record usage. Once again, subject matter experts and the team as a whole must be sensitive to these inherent biases and varying perspectives that are a natural part of team dynamics. Some influencers may be very set in their opinions and not be very knowledgeable concerning the innovation present in electronic document management systems; further these influencers may not understand the need for the EDMS as the LHR. Often the HIM manager can help educate this group of stakeholders and point them to resources.

This group of influencers may include clinicians, such as physicians and nurses, who are used to documenting and accessing records in a certain way; or risk management or compliance staff who may be concerned about changes in policy like the destruction of the paper records and the substitution of the electronic EDMS record as the long-term LHR. These influencers may voice their opinions strongly and become frustrated at proposed changes in the workflow to support an integrity-based legal health record. This group of influencers may even negatively challenge the acceptance of the EHR or EDMS system as a whole.

For example, clinicians may desire to view lab results in a way that compares previous episode of care results with the current results as a helpful reference to the practitioner when deciding how to best treat the patient. However, if this display replaces the ability to only view those lab tests and results performed with the current episode of care, and the coding team cannot differentiate past test results from current tests, inaccurate codes, charges, statistics, billing, reimbursement may be impacted. Clinicians may also desire to keep records for time periods more extended than actual retention standards. The long-term cost of this extended storage, and the labor needed to process release of information requests, may not be recognized by practitioners, but can become an obstacle for the overall organization. These strong and potentially negative reactions should be anticipated and handled as part of change management strategy through frequent communication and education as to the benefits to workflow and efficiencies in the management of electronic records.

All groups of stakeholders should be involved in the project as early as possible, get issues out on the table through open discussion, and attempt to reach a common ground based on shared beliefs and outcome goals. As the subject matter experts intervene with education and awareness and focus on the goal of transition, the project manager can successfully navigate through the culture and approval processes to move the project forward.

⊙ Steering Committee

Once the stakeholders have been identified, the appointment of a steering committee to lead the EDMS project is the next step in a successful implementation. The steering committee will certify that the change management element, so critical a part of the adoption process, will be handled with the emphasis and importance it deserves. It also ensures that the implementation team has a champion, such as an administrator or other organization leader assigned to it, as well as a forum through which to manage project activities.

Consider the following sample list of individuals that may be selected to compose an EDMS and LHR steering committee:

- ⊙ Health information management director, manager, or other representative who serves as a project leader
- ⊙ Information technology officer or manager
- ⊙ Risk management director or manager
- ⊙ Chief compliance office or manager
- ⊙ HIM systems analyst
- ⊙ Nursing representative, who may be an individual with a title such as informaticist, systems analyst, or nurse educator
- ⊙ Forms management representative or clinical documentation improvement specialist
- ⊙ Telecommunication, physical facility, or plant infrastructure specialist (as needed)
- ⊙ Medical staff representative—physician HIM liaison
- ⊙ Ancillary department representative (as needed), such as radiology, laboratory, pharmacy, emergency department staff

⊙ Chief financial officer or other executive champion

⊙ Facilitator, who may be an internal or external consultant contracted for this purpose

Develop and utilize a charter to guide the group in its mission relative to EDMS/LHR; the charter will be dependent on the stage of implementation and goals of the facility. The list of members and the focus of the team may evolve over time, depending on whether the project is in early stages of selection, mid-phases of configuration and design specifications, implementation, training, or post-implementation.

Figure 4.2 is a list of typical tasks that members of the EDMS steering committee may potentially work on either as individuals or in groups.

Figure 4.2   EDMS steering committee tasks

Initial Tasks:
- Defining a charter for the team
- Determining members and roles
- Determining potential involvement of consulting expertise
- Creating the current process map for existing workflow
- Identifying problem areas in current workflow including backlogs, user dissatisfaction, work inefficiencies, and data integrity concerns
- Creating a desired best practice process and workflow map
- Creating a gap analysis between current processes and desired best practice process maps
- Create list of requirements or request for proposal (RFP) for the type of EDMS needed
- Begin work on data dictionary until completed
- Begin work on forms inventory until completed
- Begin work on legal health record inventory until completed
- Review current record retention standards
- Review current legal health record definition or create LHR definition manual
- Research current EDMS vendors and invite for interviews and demonstrations

Preimplementation:
- Interview or visit customer sites for EDMS validation
- Select final vendor and receive final pricing
- Prepare budget and timetable for approval and implementation planning
- Once approved, notify vendor to begin implementation planning
- Plan for space acquisition or remodeling and redesign to accommodate changes

- Evaluate current job descriptions, roles, and pay scales relative to workflow changes
- Create productivity and quality standards for EDMS tasks
- Begin recruitment or interviewing for staff changes or new roles needed
- Send out regular communications and updates across facility
- Purchase and test equipment
- Configuration and system set-up
- Create test and live environments
- System testing until approval
- Create reconciliation process
- Select key data indicators for measuring performance objectives
- Prepare training materials
- Update or create new policies and procedures
- Conduct orientation or batch training sessions for preparation for go-live

Go-live/Ongoing—Postimplementation:
- Create designated team for assistance during go-live
- Train one-on-one for clinicians and providers upon go-live
- Create triage process for problems
- Collect ongoing productivity and quality data for indicators
- Verify there is an ongoing change and testing process in place for regulatory or system upgrades or changes
- Appoint designees for participation in user groups and ongoing education

The specific goals of the group may vary based on the focus of the team, however what remains the same in any well-formed steering committee is the commitment to an execution of a strategy to provide a function-rich solution that promotes data integrity, efficiency processing, and a robust workflow for health information management of the legal health record in an electronic environment.

⊙ Health Information Management Involvement

Health information managers have a tremendous responsibility in healthcare facilities as the guardians of the legal record. Whether acting in an executive or staff capacity, their unique blend of clinical, administrative, financial, analytical, and technical skills make these professionals high in demand. An important part of the human dynamics that makes projects successful is ensuring the correct subject matter expertise is brought to the table to help lead these activities. Implementing an EDMS project is a perfect example of such a project in a healthcare facility and understanding how to become better involved or understanding the lack of involvement is a key to guaranteeing the success of a complex technology project.

In a May 2013 article, the author points out that the "US Department of Labor expects jobs for medical records and health information technicians to jump 21 percent from 2010 to 2020" (Finn 2013). He goes on to say, "the lack of appropriately skilled talent to manage these new systems, regardless of how turnkey, accessible, and easy-to-use they may be is a real problem" (Finn 2013). With the onset of ICD-10-CM and ICD-10-PCS, the importance of clinical documentation and a method of verifying the integrity of the content of the record will continue to increase over the next few years, making a robust, yet stable LHR essential through the use of an EDMS.

With multiple projects and system changes occurring, most of which involve the HIM department, actually leading a major project such as an EDMS implementation may require hours that are beyond the absorption capacity for an already overstressed leadership team. However, a commonly discussed theme among HIM professionals is the perception of inadequate HIM leadership staff actually being involved to a great enough degree with decisions and leadership roles for system implementation. Understanding why this lack of involvement occurs and addressing strategies to counteract this issue is discussed in this section.

To reconcile the dilemma in time management, consider the following strategies as examples of how to move forward on a large implementation project:

1. Create a new job role for an HIM EDMS and LHR project manager whose primary responsibilities are to lead the project team through a successful implementation and who can transition into a long-term LHR data integrity leadership role.

2. Temporarily assign one or more existing staff members to portions of the leadership tasks necessary for a successful implementation. Temporary assignments can potentially be made by phase, with one person taking the lead pre-implementation, and another during go-live testing and implementation, and still another post-implementation for division of labor. Another division of responsibility may be by functional task providing, for example, one individual who is responsible for the forms management portion of the project, and another charged with writing policies, procedures, and job descriptions relative to the EDMS change.

3. Utilize special project hours, overtime, or temporary staffing to backfill positions so that hours can be available for assistance on the project.

4. Select and utilize expert consulting or contract hours to help facilitate the project management and provide subject matter resources as an extension of the existing HIM leadership team.

Another concern, aside from lack of resources, may be a lack of invitation for the HIM leadership to participate in the process of system selection or implementation. While this lack of participation is not necessarily an issue in some organizations, it is an unfortunate reality in other facilities, and may occur due to the system's culture or hierarchy or a lack of understanding of the workflow needs within the

HIM infrastructure. Lack of participation may also occur when assumptions are made around the need to involve the HIM leadership team when making decisions about EHR and EDMS selection and use. At times, vendor direction or instruction to an organization may inadvertently not provide for involvement of the appropriate HIM staff and, as decisions are made, they may be based on incomplete, inadequate, and even faulty information.

In yet other situations, HIM leadership may hesitate to participate and become involved due to over-commitment in other areas of responsibilities, a fear of change to the unknown, a lack of confidence in subject matter knowledge, a view that the decision is someone else's responsibility, or just an unwillingness to explore adopting technology or challenge the status quo. In an interview with the *Huffington Post*, Padmasree Warrior provided relevant advice for those facing large project challenges:

> There is no perfect fit when you're looking for the next big thing to do. You have to take opportunities and make an opportunity fit for you, rather than the other way around. The ability to learn is the most important quality a leader can have. (Bosker 2011)

Certainly the path to success, whether driven by HIM leadership, non-HIM leadership, male or female in nature, will be one filled with learning.

When experiencing some of the aforementioned challenges, consider the following tactics for the health information management professional to begin or to stay actively involved in information technology strategies. As a facility embarks on the journey of implementing an electronic health record and electronic document management system, they should consider the following points to assist in creating an information governance plan:

1. Ask to be involved. Ask to lead a project. Ask to be responsible.

2. If time-commitment conflicts prohibit involvement, ask if a representative can be appointed to serve on the committee.

3. Suggest additional resources that can be utilized to serve the committee.

4. Ask to receive minutes from a meeting and provide feedback on those minutes to the appropriate individuals.

5. Provide reference articles, resources, practice briefs or case studies to illustrate points.

6. Volunteer to research topics relevant to the committee.

7. Volunteer for other related assignments or leadership activities related to documentation strategies and the legal health record.

8. Personally get to know stakeholders, especially those with influencing authority.

9. Volunteer to provide education about HIM workflow and the legal health record.

10. Do not compromise principles for managing health information by adopting technology that does not support HIM workflow needs. Instead, follow the seven core principles of the AHIMA Code of Ethics and ask if implementing the technology:

o Promotes high standards of HIM practice

o Identifies core values on which the HIM mission is based

o Summarizes broad ethical principles that reflect the profession's core values

o Establishes a set of ethical principles to be used to guide decision making and actions

o Establishes a framework for professional behavior and responsibilities when professional obligations conflict or ethical uncertainties arise

o Provides ethical principles by which the general public can hold the HIM professional accountable

o Mentors practitioners new to the field to HIM's mission, values, and ethical principles (AHIMA 2011)

The involvement of HIM professionals in implementation is essential to the success of utilizing the EDMS as a vital component of the EHR. By continuing to work toward the goals of providing a complete electronic document management system as the legal health record within the electronic health record, the stage will be set for long-term interoperability, superior customer service to access records, and the ability to use information appropriately from continuation of care to research purposes.

⊙ Impact on Other Functional Areas of Operation

One final area of human dynamics should be considered during an EDMS implementation. Consider how this changing environment will impact other functional areas or users of the medical record. This group includes:

⊙ those who document;

⊙ those who review the record; and

⊙ those who may request reproductions—copies or electronically distributed transmissions—of the clinical record.

Keep in mind some of these individuals will not have had any experience outside a paper or hybrid use of a medical record. Others may be influenced by having had experiences dealing with a dysfunctional or fragmented environment within a patient-centered EHR and may have difficulty understanding a different approach. In either scenario, focus on understanding the impact of the EDMS as the legal health record so that expectations can be well-documented and questions answered prior to changing any policies, procedures, or workflow dynamics.

Good principles of change management such as communication, training, and participative input from individuals are important in achieving an optimal transition to new work tools and processes inherent with an EDMS. It is important to achieve continuous buy-in through education and involvement of leadership in helping the transition to occur smoothly into a Level 3 EDMS environment. Continuous buy-in can be achieved by enlisting the leadership team to help in raising awareness in others in the healthcare environment as to the importance of the EDMS in the role of patient care, workflow efficiencies, data integrity, and release of information.

The Documenters

Clinicians are the primary documenters in the patient record. In the paper or hybrid environments in healthcare, documenting may have been as simple as picking up a chart binder and writing a note. Remembering to include the appropriate elements of good clinical documentation, a date, and a signature was a manual task. Today, a lot of documentation is still completed this way.

As the paper is replaced by template-based systems, the intelligent alerts and prompts that are built into the various systems assist the documenter by pointing out gaps in documentation and even provide automatic electronic signature and date attachment so that the participant has no need to add these after each entry into the record. These alerts and prompts create an automated ongoing audit trail that is important for the end user to understand.

Clinicians are often surprised at the magnifying effect that electronic systems bring to patterns of poor documentation as a result of the audit trails. In paper record documentation systems, late entries of signatures and dates were frequently made, and it was difficult if not impossible to distinguish an entry made at the time of completion from one made months later. With an EDMS or an EHR, the recording of the date and time provides immediate information that displays the concurrency or tardiness of any entry. Entries that are out of order chronologically can also be easily identified.

A 2009 study conducted in Austria on 5,555 episode-of-care encounters observed that "physicians spent 26.6 percent of their daily working time on documentation tasks" versus time devoted to direct patient care or other activities (Ammenwerth and Spötl 2009). Although a more recent study on this has not been done, if you query physicians today, some of them are reporting even greater percentages of time spent on documentation instead of direct patient care activities.

An EDMS provides the ability to review and complete all outstanding documentation from a single source at the same time to clinicians responsible for documentation in the medical record, thus resulting in time savings and an efficient workflow. An EDMS also provides the added benefit of being able to track documentation in a centralized workflow software system so that deficient and incomplete patterns of documentation can be monitored based on patient discharge date statistics per physician.

The process of a clinician being able to view all documentation from a single source is in opposition to a configuration of a fragmented EHR, which requires electronic signature or completion within each individual source system after the original creation of a note. In a combination system, the process of creating a source document within the EHR portion of the system can provide the documenter with the ability to complete and sign a notation but then transfer the document, signature, and date to the EDMS for permanent storage, revision, modification, and archive purposes. If left unauthenticated at time of discharge, the signature portion of the document that is missing would then be completed within the EDMS. The view of the documents or completion screens of the various systems present themselves seamlessly to the clinician, who doesn't need to recognize the system in which they are documenting, as long as the signature can get applied. Due to today's graphical user interfaces (GUI), switching between systems for advanced functionality and workflow tools can work effectively to help bridge the gaps between an EHR and EDMS.

If additional documentation is appended to the core medical record, no question arises on the versioning or the piece of software that provides a controlling source for the original documentation within the system. All completion tasks can be handled concurrently or retrospectively within the EDMS deficiency analysis workflow software. This software provides the ability for the documenters to remotely and electronically review and complete all missing, incomplete, or unsigned records or to answer questions in this process.

In the majority of facilities actively utilizing document management system technology, the transfer of the electronic documents into the EDMS from the clinical documentation system occurs at point of discharge so that, until that time, the source system within the EHR owns the document and a complete packet of discharge output is created as the legal health record. This principle will play an important role in building the backbone of future workflow for the EHR and will be further discussed in chapter 9, where paths to the future in health information management are discussed.

Release of information functions can be done even on a partially completed record, regardless of the stage of completion and without the risk of a dynamic versioning conflict in documentation as long as the record's stage of completion is identified to the requestor. For example, if the record is missing a lab report, it should be noted that the lab report is still outstanding at the time of record release. Only when a medical record is considered *complete and final filed* should the person who fulfills a request for information not provide a disclaimer as to the stage of completeness.

The concept of identifying all documents within a single episode of care as complete or incomplete during the release of information process is a key principle and best practice for maintaining data integrity in the legal health record and providing for risk mitigation.

The Reviewers

The reviewers of the medical record are the internal viewers or users of the medical record rather than external requestors. These individuals have a legitimate need or right to access documentation in the record. Examples of these legitimate needs are:

- ⊙ Performing routine work such as reviewing the chart for the purpose of coding the diagnoses and procedures
- ⊙ Investigating a specific patient-related occurrence such as the administration of medication
- ⊙ Tracking a specific employee occurrence like the length of time spent with a patient
- ⊙ Auditing for record content, such as measuring the completeness of orders
- ⊙ Monitoring employee performance such as reviewing the elements in a documented operative report to ensure a proper count of surgical sponges were removed during a procedure

⊙ Reviewing the quality of the record documentation or patient care itself when, for example, reviewing documentation relative to an anesthesia reaction

⊙ Performing a clinical research study as part of an investigative review board that is charged with approving an external oncology clinical trial

An EDMS creates great efficiencies for these types of reviewers because the users are not limited to physically retrieving the paper file as they would be in an all-paper environment. In an EDMS, simultaneous access to the same encounter of care is available as long as users have access rights to the data. Reviewers also are not encumbered by the limitation of an EHR that may require searching within various source systems for different components of the record that are not in an easily accessible version, not available to a certain user because of role and access restrictions, or not eligible for review because the documents are still in an incomplete or pending phase. Within an EDMS, no question exists as to the stage of completion of the medical record, and it can be electronically locked for access based on privileges and role-based rules that may limit any unintentional potential privacy and compliance violations.

Using an EDMS, reviewers see great benefits in workflow because the request process for chart review is typically simplified and aided by intricate indexing of each document within the record. Specific types of radiological exams or nursing teaching plans are clearly identified in the EDMS index for each specific episode of care. The more detailed the indexing within the EDMS, the better the search capabilities of the system for the reviewers. For example, if the index is cross-referenced with the master patient index (MPI), demographic variables such as length of stay, discharge dates, and zip codes as well as diagnosis and procedure codes can assist with such functions as cancer registry case finding, record retrieval for quality reviews, and other record requests that require entry of specific matching criteria to determine the correct record retrieval for internal users. In fact, record retrieval can be streamlined for all who need ongoing record review, retrieval, and follow-up as part of their daily work activities.

Similar time savings can be found for a variety of review purposes. If the record is cross-indexed against variables such as charge entry, retrieval of medical records can become even more granular and the possibility of linking the complete medical record to discrete data indicators such as those available in a data warehouse can further assist when identifying retrieval criteria for medical record requests. Functionality will vary with specific EDMS software solutions, but in a best practice environment, the act of requesting a record review will provide a means to indicate search criteria so electronic records within the EDMS can be queued for immediate review purposes. The more sophisticated systems will allow retention of review criteria for repeat reviews set up on date cycles for key requestors.

The following list demonstrates some examples of the creative ways that record indexing can be linked to the EDMS for retrieval and review purposes for various functions, audits, and departmental needs.

⊙ Pharmacy: Records that show adverse effects to medications, poisonings, or other drug reactions based on codes linked with records.

⊙ Patient Relations or Risk Management: Records that show falls, use of restraints, complications, repeat emergency department patients, litigation pending files, readmissions for the same diagnosis within a specified time period, or length of stay outliers.

⊙ Medical Staff: Records that show more than a specified number of consultations, length of stay outliers, delinquent record trends by type of deficiency such as delayed radiology readings or missing operative reports by time of discharge, total charge outliers, complications, or specialized studies on a certain procedure or diagnosis.

⊙ Nursing: Unsigned verbal or telephone orders post discharge, patients transferred in or out of the unit, late addendums to the record.

⊙ Clinical Documentation Improvement: Number of queries generated concurrently as opposed to retrospectively or records where the final paid DRG was different than the original DRG.

⊙ Cancer Registry: All oncological diagnoses with pathology reports.

⊙ Pacemaker Registry: All records where a pacemaker was inserted.

Proper planning and preparation of indexing detail will assist retrieval of the complete record for reviewers, and the EDMS can provide an audit trail of reviews based on the requested queues as an added impact benefit.

The Requestors

For purposes of this chapter, the term *requestor* refers to external requestors of the patient record, such as clinical practitioners who have not historically treated the patients but may do so in the future as part of continuity of care. Requestors may also be researchers, third party payers or other reviewers and auditors, students, attorneys, and patients themselves. For the most part, these requestors provide requests that would be processed as part of the release of information (ROI) workflow within the HIM department that is supported by the EDMS workflow software application.

The ROI process is probably the area that experiences the greatest amount of impact and efficiency as a result of implementing a Level 3 EDMS solution. In a best practice environment, the legal health record can be assembled immediately after discharge, with no question as to versioning or stage of completeness. The tracking available to the HIM staff when processing a request should be able to document the request, including a copy of the physical or electronic request document, and indicate the details of what is disseminated to the end user.

The information is most often disseminated via printed copy, facsimile, generation of compact disk (CD), or viewed and printed via a self-accessible web portal. Control for access is determined by legal regulation and organization policy, as is the charging process. Sophistication of ROI functionality within EDMS systems is a key reason why the EDMS is used as the legal health record instead of a generic EHR. The tools of an EDMS should accommodate disclosure tracking, whether in the case of an external review agency such as the Office of the Inspector General (OIG) or a patient looking for information about the history of his or her own care.

Advanced functionality such as the ability to track charges associated with billing and release of information may be included in the EDMS solution, as well as an ability to electronically share information with other organizations such as the Social Security Administration, insurance carriers, or health information exchanges (HIEs). Facilities are beginning to utilize universal authorizations for information release in certain situations, and the ability to associate the whole episode of a single encounter, without having to create separate documents (typically PDF files) as duplicate images of what is released, can create significant time savings for the HIM staff.

In best practice settings, other enterprise-type documents that are applicable across multiple patient care admissions or encounters such as advanced directives forms, driver's licenses collected at point of registration, or insurance cards for billing purposes may also be stored within an EDMS and associated with all episodes or with a single episode of care within the MPI. This approach provides an ongoing positive benefit and impact for both the patient and related departments involved with the processing of these types of materials, which may be unwieldy to handle or difficult to locate in the routing EHR environment or health information system (HIS).

As request needs mature over time, access via an electronic portal will continue to grow. The EDMS can serve as the centerpiece in communicating with portals and provide a protective level of security, assuring release of a complete or abstract medical record without a concern for the dynamic nature of the patient-centered EHR. The patient-centered EHR was designed for longitudinal documentation over a series of encounters instead of a single episode of care. Expanding access to a personal health record and providing the ability to incorporate key historical documents such as the transcribed history and physical or a cumulative lab result summary can be apportioned out of the complete LHR and made accessible within the portal for viewing by patients and other requestors within these portals.

For all individuals involved in electronic medical record documentation—the documenter, the reviewer, and the requestor—can benefit from changes that the EDMS provides in terms of workflow simplification, document audit and disclosure trails, and automate the request and receipt process for access to the records.

 From newly created or rewritten job description due to emerging industry roles and productivity and quality monitoring standards, the implementation of an EDMS as a best practice model for the legal health record allows the HIM department to move from a file-and-retrieve function to a true information provider and data integrity champion of the healthcare team.

⊙ Best Practice and Innovation Takeaways

Best practices in the human component of the electronic health record management (EHRM) environment are unique to the culture, size, and infrastructure of each individual healthcare organization. However, as unique as these practices may be, they share one thing in common—they take the workflow and needs of the staff into consideration as they bring together human resources to support the growing technologies and complexities that come with HIM functions in the electronic health record.

By putting the structure of a steering committee in place, by involving the right cross-mix of professionals, and using external subject matter experts where needed, an organization is more likely to succeed when implementing any system.

Drawing from the workflow examples discussed in chapters 2 and 3, the process mapping that was used to provide a plan for changes in workflow can be correlated to the planning a steering committee of stakeholders does to create a roadmap in project success for the EDMS as the legal health record.

Centralized approaches in record management, reduction in redundant work processes, realignment of staff expectations and roles, and a properly designed physician department layout with carefully chosen equipment to support the technology go a long way toward a smooth operation. The planning cycle should take approximately 6 to 18 months from the start of the initiative to build a robust legal health record through use of EHRM principles, and the time to start for any facility that is struggling with data and document integrity is now.

In the next chapter we continue discussing the importance of the human element of EDMS by exploring other productivity enhancements and workflow impact factors at the more granular level of day-to-day processing in the HIM department.

REFERENCES

American Health Information Management Association. 2011 (October 2). Code of Ethics (revised and adopted by AHIMA house of delegates). http://library.ahima.org/xpedio/groups/public/documents/ahima/bok1_024277.hcsp?dDocName=bok1_024277

Ammenwerth, E. and H.P. Spötl. 2009. The time needed for clinical documentation versus direct patient care: A work-sampling analysis of physicians' activities. Institute for Health Information Systems, UMIT—University for Health Sciences, Medical Informatics, and Technology Tyrol, Hall. Austria. http://www.lina-schwab.de/Publikationen/z55.pdf

Bosker, B. 2011 (October 27). Cisco tech chief outlines the advantages of being a woman in tech. *The Huffington Post.* http://www.huffingtonpost.com/2011/10/27/cisco-chief-technology-officer-woman-in-tech_n_1035880.html

Finn, T. 2013. How Does Healthcare IT Re-Invent Itself Amidst a Serious Skilled Labor Shortage? Healthcare Matters. http://hcmatters.com/2013/05/how-does-healthcare-it-re-invent-itself-amidst-a-serious-skilled-labor-shortage/

Stewart, E. 2014. Personal communication with author.

Chapter 5

Job Roles, Productivity, and Quality Management for Electronic Document Management Systems

When investing in new technologies, changes in workflow can influence the productivity and quality of the work processes supporting document management and the electronic health record (EHR). These changes subsequently impact both staff and management within and external to a health information management (HIM) department. This chapter focuses on evolving job roles, staff productivity, outsourcing functions, and quality considerations within the HIM department, particularly related to the prepping, scanning, indexing, and quality review functions, as well as other clerical, technical, and leadership roles and include a review of key staff processes used to support an EDMS application.

⊙ Overview

Electronic document management systems (EDMS) as a component of the EHR typically do not function as a standalone piece of software. These systems are integrated into the larger infrastructure of the health information system (HIS) environment within a healthcare facility. The EDMS is a vital software component of the EHR that allows users to benefit from true workflow and automation efficiencies. Other software applications that are also part of the EHR may include systems such as clinical documentation software, order entry templates, master patient index systems, and other charting applications that together generate the full content of the EHR. As a result of this mix of eclectic software and systems unique to a single facility, the variations from vendor to vendor in format and functional design, site-specific file configuration, and even the version of the software will influence productivity and quality distinctly within the EDMS. There are, however, similarities that are common to all EDMS and EHR systems, starting with productivity and quality.

73

Key points in time to check productivity and quality within the EHR are prior to implementation of an EDMS, during the implementation, and post implementation at regular intervals, such as monthly or quarterly based on an individual organization's needs. Quality and productivity measures are the results of human participation and contribution into processing or managing the content of clinical documents. To build efficient productivity and high-level quality into the workflow processes surrounding the EDMS, one must start with thoughtfully designing new and changing current job roles within the HIM department. Once these job roles are clearly identified, the correct staffing volume, and skill set is provided to support the implementation, key performance metrics can be created. The development of key performance metrics can be identified prior to implementation to gauge success and monitored throughout the implementation process to gauge gradual or significant improvements. Eventually, variations between individuals or facilities can be tracked through performance indicators to help a facility monitor its success.

⊙ Changing Job Roles

Just as the work environment and workflow processes change with the introduction of an EDMS as described in chapters 2 through 4, the job roles for individuals who are the primary users of the system also will go through significant change. Thoroughly understanding these changes is important in order to rewrite job descriptions and work standards, match these positions to a proper pay grade, and recruit individuals or retrain existing staff so that the staff has an appropriate skill set to support the EDMS.

Following is a list of key job roles within the HIM department as well as job roles external to HIM. The job roles reflect changes that are typically experienced function by function when transitioning from paper or a hybrid environment into using a Level 3 EDMS as the legal health record (LHR).

Health Information Management Clerical Roles

In the paper and hybrid environments, clerical positions are the entry-level positions that typically perform chart pick up, medical record folder creation, report filing, report refiling, medical record filing, chart retrieval, file purging, and other miscellaneous tasks.

Chart Pickup

Chart pickup will continue in the EDMS environment. In fact, the need to pick up or collect all printed paper discharge records from patient care areas becomes more important with the use of an EDMS, since availability of the LHR in an electronic environment depends on rapidly scanning and processing paper documents. In addition to the routine tasks associated with reconciling the receipt of discharged patient records, electronic reconciliation of any computer output laser disk (COLD)-fed documents that get integrated into the EDMS will also be occurring at time of patient discharge.

Medical Record Folder Creation

In the paper world, charts that are collected from the patient care areas upon discharge are typically put into a traveling file folder once they arrive in the HIM department.

This folder would usually be labeled with the patient name, encounter number, dates of discharge, and medical record number. A permanent folder is later created once record processing has been completed and the record is ready for permanent shelf storage and filing with labels identifying the name, number, or year of visit for each new discharge encounter. As a best practice, some facilities create this permanent folder as the traveling folder. Creating these folders or even using folders is no longer necessary with the digital documents and folders within an EDMS environment, thus creating cost savings for the organization or provider, even though portions of the health record may still be created or printed onto paper, and then collected by the HIM staff upon discharge. Some facilities continue to use temporary folders for the traveling records that are still in a process phase for EDMS as a way to keep the papers separated prior to any scanning. The volume of paper records fluctuates from facility to facility based on the degree of automation that is in place, but paper records are not expected to disappear completely from the EDMS process at any time in the near future. Paper will be eliminated only upon implementation of a true complete EHR, which includes electronic generation of all health data and information as well as print restriction capabilities such as is present in an EDMS solution.

Report Filing and Refiling

Report filing typically occurs in two areas within the HIM department whether in the paper or hybrid environment. For some organizations, the first area is the filing of printed transcribed reports into the active patient health record. The second area is the filing of loose or late reports that are received after patient discharge.

The process of filing transcribed reports into the active patient record should stop with the adoption of a Level 3 EDMS, since transcribed reports are accessible online and can be signed and edited electronically. Printed copies are no longer needed for filing in the paper health record if a digital copy exists for review online. Many facilities still print key transcribed reports, such as the history and physical or operative report, and place a copy in the health record as a point of convenience and as a backup for any system downtime that may occur for the care team.

The risk of this practice of continuing to place paper documents in the chart is that the original documents may be signed or amended by hand in paper form instead of online in the EDMS. If altered manually—such as a physician documenting an addendum on a progress note—those paper copies would have to be scanned into the EDMS instead of the digitally transcribed report file flowing electronically into the EDMS, or both reports must be maintained, either of which increase the overall EDMS cost. Scanning a document also takes up more time to complete when compared to an electronic integration. Scanning also takes up nearly double the space in the digital record when compared to the actual COLD-generated documents due to the number of bytes used in scanning when compared to digital-to-digital file transfer. For example:

> a Microsoft Word document will only require 25 kilobytes of storage space; as opposed to 50 kilobytes for the same document when scanned. The reason for this is that scanned images pick up a lot of extra information through what's called "digital noise." (Tran 2004)

In addition, filing a transcribed paper document in the patient record runs the risk of creating a duplicate paper copy that has already been printed or is already present in the EHR or EDMS. This duplication has the potential to adversely affect patient care if the clinical providers read the wrong report. Conflicting information may appear in the two different versions of the documents if a paper report is scanned and then a subsequent edit is made on either the online system or the paper report. It is considered a best practice to amend and sign all documents electronically *only* within the EDMS, as opposed to trying to sign the paper printed documents from the EHR that might be used as reference copies during the patient care encounter. If temporary paper copies are printed, use a special colored paper or a paper that indicates that these duplicate printed documents are for reference only and will not be retained as part of the LHR post discharge.

The presence of loose reports and the loose report filing process will continue in an EDMS, but the volume of late or loose reports received by the HIM department should decrease significantly in proportion to the amount of documentation that originates from an electronic source and is COLD-fed into the EDMS since fewer reports required printing. Paper reports are sorted when received, based on which are original paper documents and which are copies or COLD-based documents. The copies and COLD documents can be eliminated because they will already be present in the system, and paper copies that do not have an original electronic source will be the only reports that will require scanning into the system.

However, the process for handling loose reports will be different. In the paper environment, loose report filing consists of two steps: identifying to whom the report belongs, and then filing the report within the patient folder.

In the new environment, techniques are used to help efficiently file documents into the electronic record. Patient encounter identification data included on the report via either a printed label or printed directly onto the report through an electronic forms template in the clinical documentation system will assist in avoiding late reports and missed error correction opportunities. Any reports that do not have identification risk being excluded from becoming a part of the LHR. The EDMS system, in conjunction with the master patient index (MPI), can be used by the clerical staff to further validate any identification information in question. Electronic form processing software can produce a just-in-time digital document, personalized with the identifying information of the patient, to be used as needed within the EHR.

In the second part of loose report processing, the pages can be scanned in batches into the imaging system as long as each of the pages contains a bar code or other identifier for the form type that the scanner can use to recognize each form and sequence or index it into the appropriate patient encounter and form location. For those reports that do not contain patient identification, the data must be keyed in prior to imaging an individual report into the system so that the scanned item is placed within the proper account folder with the other documents in the specific health record.

Medical Record Filing

In many hybrid environments, where all or part of the record is permanently archived on paper, the record resides in a folder inside a filing system, usually a large file room. A paper copy of the health record still serves as the LHR and will be used to fulfill release of information requests. The clerical job role is used to perform the filing process and the refiling process of the entire health record. Many facilities have historically used a unit record system that allows multiple episodes of care to be filed within a single folder or multivolumes of folders, depending on the size of the charts in a paper-based permanent filing system.

Upon implementing an EDMS or any electronic record infrastructure, the need for storage space and related filing processes changes dramatically and immediately. The unit record concept exists in the EDMS via the master patient index-linked episodes of care. Instead of a placing the hard copy portion of the health record received during daily chart pick up in a permanent file location, these hard copies are kept in a staging and processing file organized by discharge date. This staging and processing file allows staff to have easy access to and keep track of the records by discharge date. The record retention policy (see chapter 7 for additional considerations concerning record retention) will guide the facility in determining the length of time the temporary records should be retained.

Chart Retrieval

Another clerical role may involve chart retrieval functions. In the paper world, chart retrieval was extremely labor-intensive because it required physically going to each location to retrieve charts and sometimes involved long searches if the record was in use elsewhere at the time of retrieval. In the electronic world, while chart retrieval is still a necessary function, and paper charts may still need to be accessed, the majority of records eventually will be accessed through an electronic chart request process. A common misperception in the industry is that if there is an EHR in place, there will not *be* any paper records to collect from care units. However, this is not the case, and documents such as consent forms, test results from other facilities—some hand-carried in by patients themselves, and others printed out from the EHR—will still need to be gathered and processed upon patient discharge by the HIM staff.

The modified chart retrieval process includes the steps of the requestor submitting the request and the secondary process of retrieving the record from the temporary holding or permanent file. While the submission process within EDMS allows direct query into the database and the subsequent queuing of records for review, staff may still need to retrieve older paper, microfiche, or microfilmed records and possibly request these records from off-site, remote storage locations or warehouses, including some areas that may not be owned by the provider facility. These individual record-searching processes can be time consuming and underestimated in the impact of taking on a new EDMS or EHR. Misperceptions are common concerning the amount of time this gathering of disparate and older records takes particularly when the number of different storage locations present in a single facility may be unknown.

Based on the author's experience in performing record inventories in over 50 facilities, the average hospital has between 20 to 40 different permanent record storage locations on and off-site for their permanent and active health records, across all departments. This number of storage locations is significant, and one must take into consideration the time needed to access these areas for older records when setting time standards for individuals in a chart retrieval job role.

The longer a retention policy states records must be maintained, the greater the number of records that need to be searched during release of information requests to properly fulfill the request with all available information. Larger numbers of staff will be needed to retrieve the records if a retention policy is not updated. Based on author observations and nonpublished surveys across a large number of organizations, it appears that after a period of approximately three years the volume of requests for older paper-based files will typically begin to wane due to lack of repeat patient activity, until all paper records have been purged and destroyed once the retention life has expired. Therefore it is important to define retention limits that reflect readmission patterns specific to the organization.

File Purging

File purging is the process of sorting through the permanent file to identify which patient records should be retained and which should be destroyed. The selection is often made based on the age of the record. In the paper environment, this process requires a considerable amount of clerical support time and is typically performed on an annual basis to guarantee the file system integrity. The facility will need to continue purging and destroying paper records until the retention standards have been satisfied. Purging also will be required in the electronic system and although it is not labor intensive, the retention time periods should be defined based on each type of record. It is directed by policy and performed using software utilities, typically by information technology support as opposed to HIM clerical staff.

Health Information Management Technical Roles

The primary technical roles, or professional roles as they are sometimes referred to within the HIM department, encompass the general job functions of assembly, analysis, record processing, coding, abstracting, release of information, registry work, clinical documentation improvement, and transcription. Technical roles may typically require more training or education in regard to knowledge of medical terminology, anatomy, physiology, and health information standards and principles. In some facilities, having certain certifications such as an RHIT (registered health information technician) or CCS (certified coding specialist) are required as part of the job description. Roles listed as follows are grouped into related functions most likely to be performed by a single individual within an HIM department.

Assembly, Analysis, Record Processing

The function of assembly refers to the process of sorting the discharged patient documents that comprise the health record into a certain sequence or grouped order so that it can be read sequentially to tell the story of the patient encounter.

Most frequently the record is sequenced in chronological order—think start-to-finish story book order. This start-to-finish order is generally opposite to the organization of the patient record on the active patient care units, where the most recent results and notes are placed on top of the oldest notes or sequenced first in the electronic record, which is referred to as reverse chronological order. Reverse chronological order is not an effective workflow in the HIM department and can result in missed content during review, increased labor from staff that must continually work backwards, and create more difficulty in obtaining signatures on critical documents.

Assembly, which is the act of placing document types in a specific order or sorting documents within date by document type, will continue to be important in the electronic environment when using an EDMS. But assembly primarily applies to similar documents that are repeatedly completed, such as progress notes, orders, or nurse's notes. Documents that are COLD-fed do not require date sequence sorting as the date timing may automatically perform this task upon receipt, but any documents that are paper-printed and scanned will require this sub-sort prior to scanning. The assembly process generally will get rolled into the prepping job in an EDMS environment.

Sequencing EHR content in a sectional, chronological order post-discharge encounter, similar to formats used in traditional paper records, will greatly assist end users in accurately reviewing content during their work tasks, regardless of which role they fulfill within the HIM department.

The analysis team members, who are also known as deficiency analysts or incomplete record processing coordinators, function as reviewers of the content of the EHR. These individuals perform a quality control role by reviewing the content of the record for completeness according to facility policy and external standards, and then they route the record to the clinicians to appropriately add documentation to or sign the record if it needs authentication. The analysis function is maintained after the EDMS implementation. Automating the documents within an EDMS that provides for deficiency analysis workflow software allows this function to be done rapidly and remotely—something that was not possible in the paper environment.

Record processing encompasses more than just assembly and analysis. In most facilities it includes the oversight of the incomplete record room—a place where the paper medical record files are temporarily located for a set time period so that clinicians can complete any outstanding clinical documentation post discharge. Best practices suggest that *all* paper record deficiencies be completed prior to starting the EDMS implementation. The physical incomplete record room typically is no longer needed once all incomplete records are in electronic format because chart completion can occur remotely from any location with authorized access to the users of the system. Once the remaining batch of paper records is completed, the traditional completion room can be transformed into scanning space, coding space, or clinical space, thus improving efficiencies and resulting in additional cost savings for the organization. Many facilities have retained these rooms, often including stations that can access the health record online, as a review area for both release of information staff and visiting internal or external auditors to provide oversight into these functions and to ensure appropriate privacy, security, and confidentiality of personal health information.

Prepping and Scanning

This technical function may be included as a new or modified job description that encompasses several tasks for the EDMS processing environment. Prepping the record is similar to the assembly function for the paper record, but it typically includes several more steps:

- ⊙ Receiving the paper record components that target those items that have been printed or reprinted during the patient care process.

- ⊙ Separating the documents into items that are originals that must be scanned into the system because they have not been captured electronically elsewhere, and those documents that are COLD-fed and have been captured digitally into the EHR and subsequently the EDMS. COLD documents are not rescanned unless a manual documentation entry was added to the form.

- ⊙ Repairing any tears or frayed edges, removing any staples, taping over any holes in the paper, and taping down any loose items such as telemetry or lab strips or anything attached to a shingle-style form. Documents that are not repaired may cause disruption of the digital scanning equipment.

- ⊙ Ensuring each document contains proper identification or a bar code label.

- ⊙ Confirming that groups of documents with multiple pages or dates, progress notes, and handwritten orders are sequenced in a chronological date order from oldest to newest date.

- ⊙ Disposing of any duplicate or blank forms based on facility policy.

Scanning is the act of converting a paper document into an electronic image file for long-term storage and management. This process is used for all documents received or created in a paper format so that the documents can be managed electronically and integrated with the other electronic documents in the patient health record via the EDMS. Scanning utilizes a device similar to a copy machine and can provide single-document scanning or high-speed, multiple-document scanning. Typically scanning includes:

- ⊙ Scanning single or multiple documents.

- ⊙ Checking quality images during the scanning process and rescanning if necessary.

- ⊙ Indexing the document, including mapping the document type or form number to the appropriate digital section of the LHR. Indexing will occur automatically if all document forms are identified with a forms bar code label or other identifier. If indexing is not automatic, it must be done manually by entering the document type. Indexing is used to locate the document when searching for a specific entry in the LHR.

Quality Control and Data Integrity

The quality control and data integrity roles may be new to the HIM environment with the introduction of EDMS, although the analysis role typically served to perform a similar function in the paper environment. This is the reason that analysts commonly take on quality control and data integrity roles as HIM departments evolve to using electronic sources for the maintenance of the LHR. The quality control responsibilities are best performed by a different person than the one responsible for the prepping and scanning tasks; using different individuals for each task helps to serve as a check and balance. Some of the quality control responsibilities include:

- Checking scanned documents for physical image discrepancies such as blurriness, folded edges, or unclear text
- Checking for erroneous names or health record or account numbers that may have happened because a scanned image was attached to the incorrect patient encounter and correcting the problem or routing the issue to a manager
- Checking for sequencing issues such as out of order or missing documents
- Performing other document validity checks and identification quality reviews so that the record can be marked as finalized and made available to end users or reviewers of the health record
- Checking indexed forms to ensure that they have been appropriately and accurately indexed into the correct categories

Coding and Abstracting

Coding and abstracting functions are not new to the EDMS and EHR environments. These functions are typically done simultaneously and completed prior to or after discharge deficiency analysis depending on the organization workflow. Sequencing coding and abstracting after deficiency analysis eliminates the need for coding staff to review the record more than once if documentation is missing. Productivity is lost if coders have to reroute a record back to a physician for further dictation or completion of critical documentation.

Ensuring coders do not begin coding until a record has gone through deficiency analysis and appropriate components of the documentation necessary to code are present in the record also ensures the coders are doing the most compliant coding, which results in a robust data set that will legitimately provide for optimal reimbursement. Automatic routing systems built into EDMS workflow can electronically route discharged health records within a queue when a deficiency is fulfilled and the chart is complete and ready for coding. This electronic routing saves effort and time in the coding and abstracting process so that the episode can be billed rapidly. The abstracting process includes entering data or validating data entered by the clinician during the patient care episode. Both the coding and abstracting functions will continue to exist in an EDMS environment, so plan early to ensure that appropriate integration of other coding and abstracting software applications occurs within the EDMS or EHR software.

A change to the coding and abstracting job responsibilities that will become evident upon use of EDMS technology is the greater reliance upon the EHR, which encourages scanning of paper documents more quickly and efficiently after discharge to support the availability of the full episode of care as needed. In addition, a serious effort must be made to reduce or eliminate late loose reports so that the record is more complete at the time of coding. Finally, the organization must make a concerted effort to reduce or eliminate patient status changes and reversals, such as those that occur if the patient is designated in the MPI as an inpatient and then the HIM department receives a request to reverse the patient type to observation post discharge. While this type of situation can occur for many reasons, the root causes should be investigated and policies put into place to prevent this type of change by capturing an accurate patient status as the care is provided. These types of data element changes present unique challenges in the EHR environment and make data and document trafficking challenging due to the discrepant information trail.

Release of Information

The release of information (ROI) role and function within the HIM department is dependent on having an accessible system to retrieve, view, or print an individual patient health record. This record may be based on single or joint episodes of care or a single page or section of the episode of care. For efficient retrieval, the documents from the electronic-based episode of care must be available in a single electronic folder, similar to the paper file folder for paper documents. The logging of the request, documentation of the release, and the process of printing or electronically submitting the information is critical, as well as having a way to capture any charge policies and strategy. In environments that implement a Level 1 or Level 2 EDMS (instead of the full Level 3), the ROI function becomes extremely labor intensive because no single folder for all contents of the record exists. The ROI function in general is supported by the efficiency of an EDMS, which is designed to eliminate manual retrieval of records but this benefit can be negated if full Level 3 EDMS functionality is not implemented and separate source documents must be tracked down to aggregately compile.

Registry Work

Specific registry work involves additional data abstraction, finding records that match a certain case type, and follow-up. In a paper-based world, the registries in a healthcare setting may include the work done in a cancer registry, pacemaker registry, trauma registry or any other process involving record review and abstracting of data in single or multiple episodes of care. In any registry, there are a significant number of chart retrieval requests and a significant amount of filing and refiling. In an EDMS environment, chart retrieval requests are streamlined through automation based on using online criteria or indexed codes to search for and queue records for review by the registry team. Work queues and lists may be set up in advance, with repeating criteria, and the amount of retrieval and refiling labor greatly decreases. In addition multiple individuals may access the electronic image simultaneously from the EDMS. The shifting changes in workload in this area will cause a reevaluation of the staffing and skill levels needed in a rather dramatic fashion due to the ability to use automated tools to identify and queue records for registry processing and thus reduce the labor needed to support these functions.

Clinical Documentation Improvement (CDI)

Clinical documentation improvement specialists work either within the HIM department or outside it in another department. The CDI roles can be modified and become more efficient in an electronic environment as the EDMS accommodates the workflow of the CDI query process and feeds data and notes into the coding system. The CDI specialist is responsible for the quality of documentation in the health record to support the needs of coding and compliance functions, and the EDMS will simplify the tasks for record review. Looking at historical health record documentation as well as the current episode of care, on both a concurrent and retrospective basis, depends on access to complete documentation.

The actual process of CDI itself will be improved as more documentation becomes electronic, because the EDMS allows the CDI reviewers to read the documentation in a straight chronological book style as opposed to attempting to read the record in the fragmented segments that typically appear in clinical charting systems. Addendums as query responses can also be added directly into the EDMS as a progress note entry, captured immediately, and subsequently tagged as an active chart deficiency to encourage completion. This advanced workflow functionality is often difficult to achieve in the absence of an EDMS. The addition of other types of forms, such as a decubiti ulcer screening form created at the point of triage in an emergency department, can be recorded in the system and available for the coder to assign a *present on admission* status for each diagnosis, which must be collected by the hospital prior to billing. By reviewing the present on admission status at the same time as performing CDI, coders are saved a step in the process so that they do not have to collect this data after discharge. In fact, incorporating any concurrent documentation deficiency or collecting an item of abstracted data is one of the key benefits to utilizing an EDMS.

An EDMS may be integrated with CDI software or stand alone and serve as a reference point for the CDI specialists. Historically, CDI roles were part of the coding and abstracting functions, but in the past few years, there has been a shifting trend toward specialization. These individuals will utilize the EDMS to help promote excellence in clinical documentation in the LHR by assuring the story of the patient care episode is clearly documented and communicated.

Transcription

The transcription role includes both clerical filing and medical transcribing. Filing and refiling documents was discussed earlier in this section as a part of document dissemination, which is the clerical portion of this role. The transcriptionist job is a unique role that is partially clerical in nature and partially technical in nature; current transcriptionists serve as health language specialists who assist with document integrity during the creation of dictated and transcribed documents. The actual role of the transcriptionist, who listens to dictation and then translates and transcribes that dialogue into a print-ready text document, does not necessarily change with EDMS. The output file from the dictation, however, may be imported directly from the transcription word-processing system into the EHR and EDMS environment for access and these transcribed documents become the core content of the electronic health record. The key change involves electronic signature authentication (ESA), which can be set up to occur in one or both environments. Ensuring a consistent method for this signature process is important; in addition, a bidirectional interface should be in place to support any changes or edits to signatures that occur post-transcription. Regulating the authentication or signing of documents electronically, within an EHR or EDMS, is important since any manual signature on a printed, already transcribed document will require the additional step of scanning the document into the EDMS, which then creates a duplicate report of that document within the system This duplicate report must then be deleted or maintained based on individual facility policy.

Health Information Management Leadership Roles

Leadership roles are those job positions which have higher levels of accountability, authority, and responsibility within the HIM department. Some of the roles include direct management responsibility, and others may provide a higher level of technical expertise in a coordinator or lead type position.

Director

The director of the HIM department may be involved at a strategic level in the organization and may delegate day to day participation in the project. This person may also be responsible for coordinating or leading the educational components of EDMS to the staff. In smaller organizations, this position may also bear the primary responsibility for all of the systems analysis duties supporting the software in the HIM department, but in larger organizations, other individuals may share that responsibility.

The HIM director is often forced to be responsible, from a budget perspective, for creating a return on investment to justify the purchase of an organization's resource-intensive EHR solution, when in reality, many EHR systems do not reduce facility costs as originally suggested by the EHR vendor. In fact, the implementation of an EHR *without* a Level 3 EDMS may actually *increase* labor and supply costs instead of decreasing them due to extra efforts needed for day-to-day workflow processing. Efficiencies in workflow may not be significantly realized in an EHR environment alone, where growing numbers of HIM-related staff requests frustrate executive teams in functions such as electronic record retrieval, release of information, coding, and data integrity remediation, which tend to become more complex and painstakingly laborious in an environment devoid of a Level 3 EDMS.

Managers

In addition to changing staff roles, the management team's roles may change during an EDMS implementation. In the short term, management needs to address project-oriented tasks, including rewriting job descriptions, possibly adjusting salary scale, and paying attention to multiple education systems. A manager may also be required to plan configuration, test, work on various project teams, develop new productivity reporting logs, and set up processes for monitoring volumes, quality, and data integrity and tracking errors. Some of these activities, such as testing cases for every software system upgrade, will carry on through the life of the EDMS. Other tasks such as the initial configuration of the tables and parameters may only apply to this environment unless a major change occurs within the organization or health information system of a facility.

EDMS Specialist or Coordinator

The EDMS specialist or coordinator position is a key staff position in the implementation and long-term success of the electronic document management system. The development of a specialized position dedicated to the EDMS will help minimize time constraints of other HIM managerial staff and provide a dedicated level of expertise within HIM to move projects forward and to focus on the EDMS implementation. This person may have previously served in a role as a system analyst, lead technician, manager, or quality coordinator for the HIM department.

As a whole, the workflow and functions within the HIM Department change significantly and typically improve in efficiency and quality of output when implementing an EDMS. Awareness of these changes enables us to identify differences in job roles, leading to revisions in job descriptions and improved staff satisfaction with their positions.

See Appendix C, Sample HIM Job Descriptions, to see examples of the types of roles organizations are developing relative to EDMS systems. The AHIMA 2012 *Health information Management Staff Transformation Toolkit* provides sample HIM job qualifications, a sample Skill Gap Analysis Tool, Future State Questions for Staff Discussion, and a sample HIM Department Future State Modeling Exercise that might be helpful to review when designing new job descriptions for the EDMS and EHR environments (AHIMA 2012a). See Appendix D for these references. The information provided from the toolkit, as well as examples and samples in this book, provide guidance in structuring job descriptions to reflect the changing clerical, technical, and leadership roles in HIM as the facilities progress toward a fully functioning EHR and EDMS environment.

Roles External to the HIM Department

Any roles outside the HIM department that historically had accessed documents to review or complete the paper medical record would require additional education and training for the new replacement processes involved with an EDMS implementation so as to adjust for procedural differences due to the electronic content. External roles include facility staff and other individuals that may be outside the existing provider environment. Having a clear definition of the relationship of the individuals or entity to the provider facility is important to understand the roles and to ensure compliance with any access authorization documents for these reviewers of clinical information.

Clinicians

Physicians, nurses, and ancillary staff need to access current health records of the patients they are actively treating, as well as historical records of patients previously treated. Being able to simultaneously review and legitimately edit and sign incomplete records from remote locations are the greatest benefits of an electronic record system to these clinicians. EDMS provides the record in a single episodic, ready-to-review electronic folder, saving time for practitioners by enabling them to access the EDMS as their primary retrospective repository for the electronic health record.

External Reviewers

Students, insurance companies, government entities, attorneys, peer review organizations, state comparative databases, and accrediting agencies are just some of the examples of the types of record requestors who need access to patient health records for review purposes. The request process is simplified with an EDMS in place, and access can happen simultaneously and from a remote location. The workflow release of information system can track the disclosure access and any authorizations and exactly which items were released and the subsequent, if applicable, billing and collections.

Producing access to these documents can be completed in the following ways:

⊙ Online review at the provider site

⊙ Mailed paper copies of document or health records

⊙ Receipt of alternate media such as CD or DVD or films based on the request

⊙ Verbal read-back to the requestor after identification validation by the HIM staff

⊙ Portal access for posted documents via sign-on or link access

Whether internal or external to the HIM department, job roles will change and adapt to the electronic record environment within an EDMS, and these changes will need to be reflected in the job descriptions themselves after evaluating and documenting expected changes in workflow processes. In addition, these roles will grow in complexity as organizations implement privacy and security requirements under the HITECH Act, which significantly increases organizational responsibilities toward EHRs.

⊙ Use of Outsourcing and Consultants

It is important to include a brief mention of outsourcing and consulting because they are used in various ways in both the HIM and HIT departments. Outsourcing typically refers to the practice of hiring staffing resources to perform a function for which the staff is not directly employed by the organization. Outsourcing may be used on an interim basis to cover a temporary leave of absence, on an as-needed basis to respond to fluxes in work volumes, or as a long-term solution instead of permanently hiring someone to fill the position because of budget limitations.

Consulting services are generally used to provide strategic expertise, project leadership, and ongoing guidance to the organization when a particular knowledge gap exists. These subject matter experts (SMEs) are most helpful when utilized at the beginning of a project plan, as team leaders, and typically before final strategy decisions have been made. In some cases, consultants are brought in if a key team member is missing, if team members disagree concerning the best approach to use to move forward, to assist with vendor selection and request for proposal development, and as ongoing SMEs.

There are vendors who provide outsourcing and consulting services specific to both EHR and EDMS functions, including leadership positions, implementation staff, or clerical and technical staff to assist with prepping, scanning, and quality check processes. Some of these companies also may provide equipment or perform other supplementary services such as release of information, or paper document storage.

There are pros and cons to using outsource services for these supplemental services. With larger-scale operations, the cost of scanning labor and processes are typically minimal and easily absorbed by a healthcare facility if the facility already has invested in a full-scale EHR or EDMS. However, outsourcing may be a viable alternative if there is a labor shortage in a rural area, if volumes are unpredictable, or if staff is not available seven days per week. One of the more serious issues with outsourcing resources, despite the obvious cost associated with nonemployee labor, is the delay in turnaround time in the functions. Outsource firms often put processed records through an additional quality check and this extra step can delay turnaround times and impact responsiveness in urgent situations. Turnover can be high for outsource staff, and errors and extra time in training can also result. While these problems obviously can occur in a non-outsource environment as well, they may appear more frequently because of the HIM's lack of direct control or the temporary staff person's lack of familiarity with the health organizations when new individuals are placed in position.

Consultants typically provide a better return on investment when compared to continuously using outsourced core staff. Consulting expertise tends to be unique and may fill a niche that an organization finds difficult to recruit; similarly, consulting expertise often can serve when an organization cannot afford an individual with the experience and knowledge needed in a particular situation. Since consultants and outsourced individuals provide work without consuming benefits, and since the number of hours used is typically limited, consultants and outsourced staff are often a good investment option for the facility. In addition, having a third-party opinion from a nonemployed individual often provides objectivity to the organization during critical and strategic planning sessions.

⊙ Factors Impacting Productivity and Quality

Regardless of whether work is completed by employees or by using an outsourced service or consultant, measuring productivity and quality of staff is essential to building a solid infrastructure within the HIM and IT departments.

The prepping and scanning tasks critical to the workflow of the EDMS system during the HIM function of processing documents post discharge is an example of one of those areas. It is important to understand some of the factors that influence these tasks in order to build an environment that is productive and supports the quality of the LHR. Since the scanning task is the entry point for a significant number of documents that will be retained for an extended period of time and accessed by a large number of users, taking the time to set up these areas correctly will benefit the facility implementing the EDMS.

Prepping the record begins with pick-up and receipt of any documents that are printed onto paper, triggering a legal transfer of guardianship for the health record between the individual practitioner or clinician team providing the care and the individuals processing the record in the HIM department. Using a sign-off system to document that all records have been received is an effective way to account for and track any health records that cannot be located in a timely manner. Facilities may wish to track the trends of any missing records by service area or provider to identify ways to reduce the risk delaying records.

Once the records are received and temporarily stored and housed in the HIM department for processing, they can be accessed manually. Since electronic COLD feeds are likely to have already started flowing into the EDMS, some items will be available upon discharge, even prior to any scanning of documents. The higher the percentage of documents that are received electronically, the less manual scanning of documents need to occur retrospectively. This does not diminish the importance or use of the EDMS as the central repository for the LHR, since its main purpose—acting as the archive and management environment for the output of the health record—is still intact.

The prepping phase requires great concentration on the part of the staff working with the record. During this phase documents are sorted and initial quality checks are performed to identify those parts of the record should be scanned and those parts of the record that are already present. Identification checks are made on each clinical form to be retained in the LHR. Facilities often make the mistake of having prepping staff also serve in a dual role, typically if they are required to perform reception duties such as greeting customers or answering the phone. Distraction can create errors, and concentration in a quiet area is best suited for the prepping role. But staff performing the prepping function can also serve in the deficiency analyst role. The process of fully reviewing the record can save time later instead of repeating the review for completeness and performing other analysis processes as a separate task.

Some facilities may find they wish to have the prepping staff also perform the initial bulk scanning of the discharged records immediately after the records are prepped, typically due to the location of the high-speed scanning equipment and not due to skills competency. In a smaller environment, duality of roles is more commonplace, especially if there is only one high-speed scanner. In a larger facility where there is a division of labor, combining roles may not be as practical. However, in the larger facility, cross-training on tasks is recommended and can provide back-up relief during holidays and other times when staff is off.

The quality check or quality-control process within EDMS processing assures that the images and electronically fed documents that are received into the EDMS are clearly visible, accessible, and indexed properly. This process takes place immediately after scanning in most places, and is performed by different staff to secure checks and balances within the system. Bar codes that identify the document type, patient identification using the encounter numbers, and other key information can provide for optimal speed when scanning documents into the system. In a situation where bar codes are not available, lead sheets can be used to identify a like batch of documents, such as historical records received from other facilities, once they are sorted into chronological order. Lead sheets are then scanned into the EDMS to identify the type of document that may not contain adequate identification such as a bar code, in order for indexing directly from the form itself. Other tips to reduce the time spent prepping and scanning the documents include assuring forms follow guidelines such as being printed onto white paper instead of colored paper, using the same format for content within the documents so identifiers are located in the same position on each form, and assuring all forms are free of staples and tape, and the forms' owners are properly identified.

Just as staff have roles and productivity guidelines specific to the EDMS, the same staff will also need quality standards and requirements that apply to their job performance. These standards include turnaround time and other quality indicators.

End users such as clinicians, requestors for copies of the health record, and other staff in the provider environment benefit from a record that is complete, comprehensive, episodic in nature, and accessible in a timely manner. Assuring that records are available as quickly as possible after discharge and processed accurately are key indicators of quality within an EDMS.

Quality concerns are resolved with proper training procedures that are documented in writing. Providing competency or professional development such as skill-level quizzes and ongoing education and training refreshers will assist staff in maintaining quality. With each software upgrade, a retraining session and competency quiz should be initiated for staff. If the source of the documents is of poor quality into the EDMS, address this quality issue with the owner of the source data. For more information on proper form output and process, refer to chapter 6.

⊙ Productivity Standards and Quality Measurement

A common question when adopting new technology or changes in workflow is: What is the productivity standard for a particular new task? The answer is not simple and few sources exist for this information. There are situations that negatively impact productivity, despite the myth that technology always yields improved productivity and efficiencies. For example, the creation of a new form that needs to be scanned or the adoption of another piece of software that requires additional quality checks or location searching may decrease productivity or become a bottleneck in the workflow. The way productivity is measured varies significantly from site to site, particularly in the prepping and scanning tasks described previously in this chapter due to different equipment, the volume of the records, and the types of records being scanned. Something as simple as a single folded document that needs to be unfolded during the prepping process can impact productivity.

Creating a Productivity Standard for EDMS Tasks

To determine productivity standards, an existing best-practice technique exists that can be used to create standards internally. Since there is quite a bit of site-specific variation in performing various tasks in an HIM department, this flexible, best-practice technique can be used for a facility that has an EDMS in place to create its own standards that combine site-specific values and industry best practice standards. The leadership of the HIM department should set up a mechanism for measuring productivity and collecting the data that can show the trends in terms of volumes and impacting issues. Figure 5.1 defines steps to follow to create a reliable productivity standard for your EDMS functions.

Figure 5.1   EDMS productivity steps

☑ Define the tasks and steps to include in a single workflow process. For example, the scanning step may include:

   a. Retrieving the documents and charts to be scanned.

   b. Filling out header information on a lead sheet for batch scanning.

   c. Inserting documents into the scanner.

   d. Verifying documents on-screen to confirm accurate placement, image rotation, content clarity and completeness, such as four pages received of four pages scanned.

   e. Validating that all scanned images display patient-identifiable information.

   f. Checking that all scanned pages are indexed to the proper document and section categories within that health record for a specific episode of care.

   g. Recording the number of images scanned for productivity tracking purposes.

   h. Marking the documents for destruction date.

   i. Refiling or transferring the documents to the quality control specialist for review.

☑ Using a stopwatch, record the exact time to complete all of the tasks and multiply that value by the number of records to be processed (minimum 30 recommended). Repeat this process on several different days and, if possible, using several different staff.

☑ Capture the average of this data as internal standard. Use consistent methods of capture based on industry standards such as a given amount of minutes per health record or so many health records or forms per hour. Verify this standard's measurement is the same, regardless of whether the standard is internal or external.

☑ Search external references for written productivity standards relative to the function in question, such as document scanning. For example, search professional associations such as American Health Information Management Associations, American Record Management Association, specialty groups, social media groups, vendor standards groups, and technology company client forums or user groups that specialize in working with EHR and EDMS. Capture the average of this data as applicable as the external standard.

☑ Average the internal and external standards.

☑ Create a range from approximately 5 percent below this standard to 5 percent above this standard. For example, if the average is 1,200 documents per hour to be scanned, the standard range for acceptable production would be calculated to be between 1,140 to 1,260 documents per hour. In this way, variations and rewards for productivity as a performance measure can be associated with various staff.

☑ Use external consulting expertise to conduct a productivity study if time is a constraint in developing these standards throughout a department.

It is important to ensure employees have a method to record productivity. While some software programs collect data automatically, best practices suggest that you create a way to track and measure productivity on a person-by-person, individual reporting basis using a productivity tracking form that you develop.

See figure 5.2 for an example of a Productivity Tracking Tool that can be used by the EDMS staff. This particular example supports collecting data on the prepping, scanning, and quality indexing functions so that leadership staff in HIM may collect and track data. Of note is the 20 percent downtime element introduced within the spreadsheet. Facilities often include nonproductive time allotted for staff to perform other functions, take a lunch break, and so on during each working day, and adjust time accordingly on the productivity reporting tool. A more detailed productivity tracking sheet for just scanning functions is included in chapter 9 as this is often a difficult area to track properly with any detail.

The process for collecting productivity statistics on a task must be clearly documented or the data received from various staff members will be inconsistent. For example, to measure a stack of forms to be scanned, one can choose to measure by the number of sides or images of the documents, by the number of pages of documents, before the removal of COLD documents, after the removal of COLD documents, or estimate in inches, just to name a few variations. Regardless of the measure chosen, it should be consistently applied for all task measurement across all employees.

General Record Processing Production and Quality Standards

The following are suggested best practice production and quality standards and indicators to monitor for the overall EDMS as well as for individual employee performance.

Figure 5.2   Sample productivity tracking tool

EDMS SAMPLE PRODUCTIVITY TRACKING TOOL

Task	Metric	Site 1	Site 2	Site 3	Site 4	Site 5	Site 6	Site 7	Site 8	Site 9	Site 10	Site 11	Site 12	Site 13	Site 14	Site 15	Site 16	Site 17	Site 18	Site 19	Av Std
Prep	Images/Hr		305	750	375	1400	1100	420	800	800	800	450	450	500	400	175	see list	1000	1313	700	690
Scan	Images/Hr	2000	670	2500	625	2500	4200	1800	2000	2500	3000	1500	1200	2000	1800	175		3000	4500	4000	2221
QC/Index	Images/Hr	700	280	750	935	2100	2100	500	500	700	800	720	750	1700	800	175			616	700	895
Index Alone	Images/Hr						760											800			
QC Alone	Images/Hr							1850													
QA	Images/Hr																				
Image/Inch				125		225			200												
Prod Time/Hrs						8				7.5	6.5										
Analysis/Hr Inpatient										10	8										
Analysis/Hr ED										19											
Analysis/Hr OP Sx											16										
Analysis/Hr OP											90										

Adapted Courtesy of HIXperts_Productivity Tracking Tool, W.K. McLendon, RHIA

1. Less than 1 percent duplicate health record numbers or accounts numbers generated

2. Less than 1 percent unidentified forms or documents within the health record

3. 100 percent of all COLD documents reconciled including those sent versus received in a volume count comparison

4. Less than 1 percent late or loose reports received by HIM department post discharge

5. 100 percent of all records received within 24 hours of discharge

Turnaround Time and Quality Standards

Use the following best practices as guidelines for turnaround time quality standards, which should be maintained seven days per week:

1. All health records prepped and scanned within 24 or less hours of patient discharge from facility to ensure rapid availability to clinicians who may need to access for patient care, particularly in cases of readmission to a facility.

2. All health records electronically analyzed within 48 hours of patient discharge from facility to ensure coding of the records begins no later than the second to third day post discharge, and to provide the least gap possible from discharge to prompting deficiency completion of the record for the clinicians.

3. All health records coded within three to five days post discharge, if pertinent documents are complete within the record. Typically, most facilities have a three to five day post discharge hold on account billing due to pending late reports and charges cumulated from the episode of care.

Individual Quality Performance Standards

Use these best practices as guidelines for individual quality performance standards:

1. 100 percent accuracy in scanned image and identification content. The point of the quality review process is to assure 100 percent accuracy in image content. So eventual 100 percent accuracy is not something that would be difficult to achieve.

2. 95 percent accuracy in document indexing. This accuracy level is a typical one observed in HIM departments. While the goal may be 100 percent, 95 percent is a more realistic measure.

3. 95 percent accuracy in overall coding and abstracting. Data integrity is crucial to good information. While 95 percent may seem low, it is typically the most common practice seen in coding audits conducted by various consulting firms.

Certifying quality standards and productivity standards are in place within an organization that is using EDMS to manage electronic health records assures the highest user satisfaction and provides for integrity of the content of the archived LHR.

⊙ Best Practices and Innovation Takeaways

There are various factors throughout the organization that will impact the productivity and quality of the LHR. When implementing an EDMS, a key to good productivity and improved quality of the LHR is to support efficient handling of the documents, both paper and electronic, through use of best practices.

The following is a top 10 best practice list of steps to be completed prior to an EDMS implementation; following these steps will help optimize the system's use and innovate success from a productivity and quality perspective.

☑ Verify all forms that are part of the health record contain accurate bar code identification for form type to allow automatic indexing during scanning.

☑ For those documents received externally that do not include bar codes for indexing, use document leader sheets, which act as header forms to be scanned prior to a document or series of documents.

☑ Confirm that an up-to-date prepping list is available for HIM staff identifying the documents to be scanned and imaged and the documents that will be integrated electronically via computer output laser disk (COLD) process.

☑ Reduce the use of staples and tape within documents to avoid scanning issues. Ensure that telemetry and other strips completely adhere to forms as they are generated during the patient care process to avoid spending time to fix post discharge.

☑ Using a separate staff position, check the quality of images and indexed content immediately following the scanning process to guarantee integrity of the data.

☑ Certify that 100 percent of all documents are flowing into the EDMS from any clinical documentation or electronic health records system in place to prevent searching for segments of the record in different locations. The reconciliation process also helps to confirm the completeness of each individual episode of care.

☑ Provide a single source for managing all clinical record deficiencies, including incomplete records processing. A single source for clinician completion helps provide efficiency to users as well.

☑ Invest in desk scanners for individuals handling loose or late reports, and high-efficiency, high-speed scanners for batch processing. State of the art equipment means saving time for staff.

☑ Use a scan-forward philosophy for patients readmitted to a provider facility. A scan-forward philosophy provides that any paper records be scanned and indexed for access within the EDMS as opposed to filing and refiling and retaining historical paper records. This approach means not scanning older records, but instead scanning previous records only when requested for review at the time of a subsequent encounter of care. Outguides may be used as a placeholder in the file system to indicate the scanned forward record absence.

☑ Destroy paper health records within 90 days of scanning and processing within the EDMS to avoid dual handling and searching and costs associated with the storage and maintenance of the temporary paper record.

Many aspects of paper record management influence job roles and day-to-day workflow in the HIM department. The next chapter focuses on the primary key to success for any EDMS or EHR—effective forms management. Excellent documentation results from well thought-out document design and controls as healthcare organizations prepare for the future with new classification systems, advancing software technology, and computer-assisted coding.

REFERENCES

American Health Information Management Association. 2012a. *AHIMA Health Information Management Staff Transformation Toolkit*. Chicago: AHIMA.

American Health Information Management Association. 2012b. *Document Management and Imaging Toolkit*. Chicago: AHIMA.

McLendon, W.K. 2014. HIXperts_Productivity Tracking Tool. In communication with author.

Tran, T. 2004. The Basics of Document Sizing. http://www.supportingadvancement. com/records/document_imaging_sizing/document_imaging_sizing.htm

Chapter 6

The Importance of Forms Management

Just as workflow is the most important component of a fully functional electronic document management system (EDMS) for healthcare facilities, forms management is the single most important task in both implementation and long-term maintenance of a successful legal health record (LHR) within the EDMS or electronic health record (EHR).

The terms *forms*, *documents*, *reports*, and *output* are referred to synonymously when discussing the visual presentation of clinical notes and results within a patient health record, whether it is in paper form or electronic format. One often finds hundreds of different forms used within the course of health record documentation in a single healthcare organization.

⊙ Overview and History

In the paper medical record, forms primarily consisted of printed document templates that were used to record mostly handwritten information. Other documents would be transcribed within word processing systems, just as they are today, but printed instead of delivered electronically into an EHR or EDMS. The form templates would be either generic-style templates that were printed onto individual pages—single-ply or multi-ply paper—or customized templates that were created specifically for a facility by a print shop. External vendors would supply the generic templates for purchase or would typeset and print the customized templates. Print shops or graphics departments were commonly established in larger facilities to do much of the design and printing inside a facility to avoid external fees. With word processing and personal computers used increasingly in healthcare in the 1990s, modification of these customizable forms became more common and affordable even to smaller facilities, many of which started handling these documents in-house.

As computerized documentation solutions within various health information systems (HISs) and electronic health record (EHR) applications began to appear and the use of personal computing grew in popularity, the ability to create just-in-time patient-personalized forms for inclusion in the electronic health record became a reality. The realization of this concept meant, for example, that a patient could be registered at time of admission to a facility and a demographic fact sheet that contained personal details about the patient specific to an episode of care could be printed; this demographic fact sheet would contain all of the data that was entered directly into the patient's registration form during the patient registration process for that encounter.

This electronic-and-printed version would also reflect the date and time of the data entry and, once printed, the electronic-and-printed version became the legal version of the record that would remain as part of the permanent, archive-ready health record once the patient discharge was completed. The collection of this date and time of entry information helped healthcare facilities track such things as turnaround time of services and compliance with documentation time protocol standards for clinicians because the data was recorded real-time as the activity occurred. The accuracy of this data became even better when the timing of data entry was automated within the EHR, creating a magnification effect that served to spotlight any late entries into the record. In the all-paper health record, when late entries were made as addenda, they often were not dated or timed and thus how late an entry actually was could not be confirmed simply by looking at the record.

In addition to the forms template concept, the data or documentation that was recorded on the form often included elements of patient identification such as the patient's name, account number, registration date, and other pertinent information relative to the specific episode of care. Bar codes were either automatically printed onto the documents or applied as labels onto the forms. Numerous sheets containing multiple bar codes with patient-identifying information could be printed and used during the patient care process to apply to any forms that did not already have a bar code printed upon them. To create the most efficient process for forms management, create as many forms as possible with preidentified bar code information on each document to avoid the costs of printing labels and the labor associated with applying them. The payoff is tremendous within the EDMS for quickly indexing the document by using the bar codes instead of using data entry; this makes the use of bar codes worth the expenditure, regardless of the mechanism used to affix the bar code to each document. Most frequently, these bar codes are designed in Code 39 standard as illustrated by the sample shown in figure 6.1, an example of a bar code that could potentially be used to indicate a one-sided consultation report, designed in December 2014.

Figure 6.1   Sample 3 of 9 bar code

Consultation_1214_1

Many of the point-of-care-oriented clinical documentation systems were designed with the input process in mind, which was designed to the requirements of clinicians who were providing active bedside support and needed to quickly document their findings and notes. The design of these systems did not consider printed output that may be needed at a later point. These EHR solutions did not produce printer-friendly documentation, since they were designed using the assumption that the health record would be archived electronically and not printed on paper. Therefore, the need for additional software solutions that could provide printer-friendly output of the health record was sought, and the need for EDMS solutions became more clearly justified over time and experience with EHR environments.

As time passed, users discovered many reasons to print a patient's health record in a paper format, even if the record was created entirely electronically within the EHR. For example, users might print health records to:

- Facilitate review for end users who may prefer paper or do not have access to a computer screen
- Mail certain documents instead of sending them electronically
- Review results in a remote location where a computer was not available
- Fax receipt of a document
- Copy the documents to distribute multiple copies
- Comply with a court deposition, subpoena, court order, or for trial litigation purposes
- Distribute copies to clinicians who wanted to retain documents in a paper health record format instead of an electronic format

The concept of formatting the output of the data or results record within these electronic templates so that the records appeared as a printed form frequently was missed in EHR design, and only fragments or portions of paragraphs or data appeared on printed output pages. For example, a record of a newborn was nine pages long as a paper record, but when it turned into an electronic document, it was approximately 80 pages long when printed. Anecdotally, facilities frequently found that printed copies of an EHR sometimes doubled and tripled the printed volume of the original paper record, so the cost of supplies such as paper and toner dramatically increased with EHR adoption. An organized design template that can be used for all documents in the health record guarantees an efficient, effective, and compliant documentation process in the EDMS and LHR.

To secure form and data integrity within health record documentation as it is used within an LHR, facilities must face the challenge of implementing a solid forms management program. A robust forms management program encompasses the following components:

- Forms inventory
- Forms committee
- Forms standardization

⊙ Forms input

⊙ Electronic document reconciliation

The rest of this chapter provides a detailed discussion of each of these areas and its impact on the EDMS system and LHR.

⊙ Forms Inventory

Taking an inventory is the process of cataloguing a set of items or assets. When deploying an EDMS solution, taking an inventory—even though it requires significant effort—is critical to the project's success. Companies that began to work with organizations to help automate patient records started experiencing delays in the projects if a proper forms inventory was not completed at the time the project was initiated.

> Formatting and preparation of documents for the EMR is the longest time line in the conversion process and must precede other project steps. If done after the fact, it can cause delays and unexpected costs. When you convert to EMR, hundreds, sometimes thousands of preprinted forms have to be redesigned, reprinted, labeled, or converted to print on demand with barcodes in order to meet the needs of the project. A good project design will provide adequate planning, solutions, and timelines for preparing and reformatting your documents. (FormFast 2014)

There are three phases to the forms inventory process:

⊙ Phase 1—Create the master list and gather a sample of all existing clinical documentation or forms.

⊙ Phase 2—Develop naming and number conventions and create standardized design elements for forms.

⊙ Phase 3—Redesign and reformat the documents in preparation for the EDMS implementation.

Phase One: Forms Collection

To complete Phase 1, perform the following steps:

1. Determine if any existing lists or partial lists of forms used in clinical documentation are available.

2. Begin to create a cumulative forms inventory list. This list would include types of documents like the following:

   ⊙ Preprinted forms ordered or received from external sources such as death and birth certificates or ambulance transfer forms

   ⊙ Forms that were printed or designed internally at the facility such as customized consent or authorization forms

   ⊙ Forms which were created or printed through an individual or department, including word processing-generated documents, such as teaching and education forms or customized progress note forms

- Forms that are produced in a mechanical output fashion from equipment like cardiac monitor tracing reports or telemetry strips
- Forms or electronically output documents that are produced electronically in another source system such as physician orders, nursing input–output charts or rehabilitation notes

3. Collect, in a master binder, a sample of each form used in the health record. Do not collect electronic copies; instead collect actual printed copies of each form, because it is important when reviewing form format to see the physical copy as it looks when printed as compared to its appearance on the graphical user interface (GUI) screen view.

4. Physically tour each department to search for additional forms that may be stored locally in a department or unit; also search storage areas for removed, unapproved, or unused forms. This search may require actually opening drawers and cabinets.

5. Collect any newly discovered form samples.

6. Organize the forms into sequential order for final archived health record storage. This sequential-order organization is equivalent to the assembly list used by HIM technicians during the post-discharge incomplete processing series of tasks.

7. Log all forms and any corresponding form identification, including name and numbers, onto the inventory you are creating.

Phase Two: Naming and Numbering Conventions

After creating a log of the current form names and numbers, many facilities choose to renumber and rename all of the forms, to create a consistent and standardized convention for the form names and ID numbers. When doing the inventory, you might find:

- Duplicate forms that share the same number
- A single form with multiple numbers assigned to it
- Several different forms share the same number
- Forms that have no number at all

A poor forms design and inventory can result in a disorganized and workflow-disruptive EHR.

To correct this situation, each distinct form should have a unique identification number. To enhance the logic of a renaming convention, a facility can renumber these forms by using a beginning letter of P to categorize all progress notes, the letter H for all varieties of history and physical type documents, and so on. Alternatively, you can use a set number to represent the type of form, the source of the form, the clinical department in which the form is used, or any other logical sorting and progression that make sense internally for the facility.

The sample log in figure 6.2 illustrates a sample forms inventory log including the elements that should be collected relative to each form.

Figure 6.2 A sample forms inventory log

Facility	List Documents that are designated as the facility's legal health record for routine legal disclosure, a pre-eDiscovery step				
Visit Type					
Document Name Data Set Report Name	**Document ID #**	**Tab or Folder**	**Location of Use**	**Source System**	**Comments**
Below are sample document names					
Advanced directives					
Emergency department					
Consents					
E-mail and messaging					
Face sheet					
Problem list					
Continuity of care data					
Diagnostic imaging reports					
Discharge summary					
Flow sheets					
H & P					
Consultations					
Laboratory reports					
Medication administration					
Minimum data sets					
Multidisciplinary notes					
Nursing documentation					
Nursing graphics					
Operative report					
Psychological assess - notes					
Physician progress notes					
Physician orders					
Bills					
Remits					
Notes					
External records					

The following is a list of elements that are key to figure 6.2:

⊙ The *document ID* is a field length to be specified by the EDMS vendor to uniquely identify each document. Examples of document IDs or names might be M1023-DS or OB-1012-SS. In M1023-DS, the M might indicate a medical form, 1023 represents a form number, and DS stands for discharge summary. In OB-1022-SS, OB could indicate an obstetrical form, 1012 could represent the date the form began being used (October 2012), and SS could indicate that the form was a single-sided form. The meanings of the different characters are facility specific and should be consistent from form to form, which explains why conducting a forms inventory across all forms simultaneously allows for a global view of the naming conventions.

⊙ The *tab or folder* refers to the section or category of the electronic chart order in the set-up of the EDMS within which a specific form or document is filed. For example, both a chest x-ray and a nuclear imaging report may be filed under a category or tab called *Radiology Results*. By assigning each form to a corresponding tab or folder, the electronic health record is maintained and the legal health record is created in a logical order.

⊙ The *location of use* column is used to designate a department, service, or provider that would be the primary user of the form. For example, Pediatrics Department, Oncology Services, or Dr. Wilson would all be appropriate entries in this field.

⊙ The *source system* is used primarily when the document or form is generated in another electronic application or when the document originates from an external vendor or is generated as the result of using a specific piece of equipment. Examples include Telemetry strips, Clinical Documentation system, and Biometric Pacemaker ID456.

Some facilities will also insert additional fields into this log such as the following items:

⊙ A *document acronym* may be added if the full name of the document is too long to place within the identification fields used on a document.

⊙ The *owner contact information field* may be added and used to identify the form's responsible owner, who will be contacted in case of issues or a need to update the information on the form.

⊙ A *start and stop date* for each form helps the facility identify when the document went into use or ceased being used.

Phase Three: Redesign and Reformat the Documents

Redesigning typically refers to modifying the content of the document, which requires multidisciplinary input, generally through a forms committee, prior to finalization of any changes. Redesigning forms can be accomplished during the inventory process or forms redesign can be handled separately from the inventory and starting before the EDMS start date.

Content changes may be appropriate under the following circumstances:

⊙ Recognizing that more than one document contains similar or the same information. For example, if the past surgical history is documented in five different locations within the record, consider eliminating any redundant fields. The benefits of these types of changes extend to performance improvement and labor savings, as well as designing a more concise documentation platform.

⊙ Recognizing that information may no longer need to be collected. For example, suppose that a facility was documenting information to collect data on a certain topic for a clinical research project, such as patient smoking history. Further suppose that the clinical study that was using this data is no longer active. One should stop collecting the data and eliminate the data field that is no longer going to be used.

⊙ Recognizing that information is not valid anymore. For example, forms may refer to equipment that is no longer used or may list a phone number or address of a clinic that is no longer in business. Delete these items to save space and time and to improve the data integrity of the document.

⊙ Recognizing that the layout of the content no longer matches the workflow. For example, if a document requires that one section be filled out before another, but the facility has changed the order in which the task occurs, the documentation fields need to be rearranged.

Reformatting documents refers to redesigning the form's physical structure and the layout of the data fields on the form. The following situations, among others, can prompt reformatting:

⊙ Lack of standardized positions such as top, bottom, left, center, and right for various data elements may need to be addressed. Variation in positioning can slow down the quality-check process. Design structure standards and data element positioning is important to good forms design.

⊙ Lack of identifying data on electronic documents that eventually need to be printed can become a problem and cause the printed output to be accidentally associated with the wrong patient or episode of care. Working with various vendors to ensure that a printed form properly identifies the episode of care and the account will help avoid errors such as wrong association.

Aside from the sheer volume of forms that must be inventoried, particular challenges in a healthcare environment are typically found that make the process of forms inventory even more difficult.

Some of these challenges include:

⊙ Obtaining existing lists of forms. Typical barriers to this task include receiving outdated lists, discovering multiple versions of the same form in use within a facility, discovering the use of the same form but with different dates or data elements, and finding no existing list of forms.

- Obtaining samples of a form. In some cases, relying on a photocopy of an existing, filled-in document or printing a completed sample record and redacting any private health information provides another way to capture the form if the original blank template is missing.

- Cooperation from other individuals and departments. Forms generation becomes very personal to an individual who has invested time and effort in the creation of a form. Hoarding forms is commonplace and results in stockpiling the form, which causes the inventory to age and become outdated and imposes an unnecessary cost to the facility. Downtime charge capture sheets, which are used infrequently but must be accessed rapidly in the case of system downtime, are a typical example of forms that get stockpiled. Although charge information is continuously updated within the facility's charge description master (CDM), downtime charge forms don't get updated as frequently. In the event of a major system shut-down, charge capture becomes a potential risk if the downtime forms aren't readily available or contain erroneous charge data because they are out of date. This problem can be prevented if the downtime charge capture sheet inventory is kept in one central area, where it can be regularly updated and maintained. Further, the centralized department is responsible for the charge capture sheet inventory, should also be in charge of distributing these downtime forms as needed and also should be responsible for the accuracy of the inventory.

In addition to these challenges, facilities frequently underestimate the time needed to actually perform the inventory and the time needed to standardize and resolve format issues discovered along the way.

Electronic systems that do not have a standard output template may have difficulty producing a concise forms output that meets minimum design standards desired by the individual organization as set by their own forms committee policy. The example that follows demonstrates a type of problem that can occur when input and output designs of clinical documentation reports are not in sync.

A hospital was being summoned to respond to a deposition. Both the HIM director and the nurse who was the primary care provider for the patient reviewed the health record and stated they were comfortable with providing testimony in this case that should support the hospital's compliance and standards of care. However, once the court case began, the nurse was asked to interpret the documentation that was enlarged in a magnified presentation for her. She responded that she had never before seen the documentation. Her statement came as a shock to the defending attorney, who had reviewed the input display screens but not the printed output with her. Effectively, the health record that had been provided to the court was in a paper version, and this paper version was so extremely different than the input screens to which the nurse was accustomed that she felt she could not answer any questions. In this case, the risk manager at the facility was concerned and was seeking assistance concerning how to address this problem. Rectifying this situation requires a redesign of input and output fields to match. Alternatively, deploying an EDMS solution for housing the LHR would easily eliminate different input and output formatting, and can avoid auditors or other reviewers questioning the integrity of the document content.

Regardless of the source of original clinical documentation, whether on paper or electronically generated, the health record must be able to stand on its own with consistent, concise, legible, and formatted printed output documentation from any applications that generate clinical content as part of the legal health record.

⊙ The Role of the Forms Committee

The forms committee is an important group of stakeholders in the healthcare facility that have a shared interest in documentation integrity for the LHR as the business record of the organization. This committee is responsible for the data capture, display, use, and approval of documentation within a healthcare entity. Forms approval processes are necessary in any type of healthcare setting.

The following individuals are recommended as participants in the forms committee.

- ⊙ Health information manager
- ⊙ Risk manager
- ⊙ Director of nursing or nurse informatics specialist
- ⊙ Representative from the medical staff or medical staff administration
- ⊙ Materials management or purchasing representative
- ⊙ Information system or technology representative
- ⊙ Ancillary care representation as needed, depending on the department involved in the discussion

Typical roles of a well-functioning forms committee include, but are not limited to, the following:

- ⊙ Approving any new forms
- ⊙ Approving any modification to forms
- ⊙ Determining the best sourcing of forms based on input from the forms, owner or creator, and considering factors such as the source of printing, where the form is stored, the form user, the form archive location and other needs
- ⊙ Coordinating with Information Technology concerning technology purchases to ensure output formats can comply with standards used at the facility; this coordination effort is particularly important for equipment-generated forms or biometric output equipment that produces clinical results such as fetal monitoring systems
- ⊙ Initiating new or revised form content in response to new legal or clinical requirements
- ⊙ Maintaining the ongoing inventory

As the committee becomes more comfortable in working through forms issues, including redesign and reformatting of forms in preparation for an EDMS, they may be able to take on larger projects such as helping to drive automation of certain key documentation processes.

⊙ Forms Standardization

Forms standardization allows documents to be handled in a consistent way, both by people, who are the consumers, users, and viewers of data, and by the technology from which the form is generated or into which the form is archived. With the exception of transcribed medical documents, standards—particularly pertaining to forms design—are lacking in the healthcare industry. The American National Standards Institute (ANSI), through its chartered subgroup, Accredited Standards Committee (ASC) X12, developed field and format definitions for transcription format and output that are widely used today, but only on a voluntary basis.

The electronic health record vendors have had continuous discussions about the importance of interoperability, which has been a large historical barrier to exchanging information. However, the lack of standards in forms field length, definition, and standardized output from the various documentation systems within the legal record is evident to anyone who has been responsible for data integrity, release, and management.

Ensuring forms standardization is the reason that using a forms committee to oversee design issues at an individual facility level is an important component in a good forms management program. The effort put into standardizing naming conventions, numbering, appearance, redesign, and reformatting prior to attempting to create a legal health record through the EDMS will result in improved productivity and easier use of the record content by clinicians and any other users.

Based on extensive consultative field observation in helping organizations transition from paper to electronic records, the author has recommended best practice standards for forms included in the LHR to include the following tips for both paper and electronic documents that may need to be eventually printed onto paper. These best practices include the following:

- ⊙ The patient identification fields or bar code field should be located on the bottom right corner of the document so it is easily visible when turning pages.

- ⊙ The title and name of the form and the date printed should be placed across the bottom margin of the documents for visibility.

- ⊙ Leave 0.25-inch margin on all sides of the form in the event copying or faxing the document becomes necessary. Margins that are preset on this type of equipment can obstruct documentation elements set too close to the paper edge, which are then not captured during the photocopy process. The top-of-page title should be used for the name of the facility or department and the title and name of the document; the title and name of the document are repeated at the bottom for clear visibility and reference when looking quickly at numerous documents.

⊙ All pages of the document should be numbered and contain the patient's basic demographic data, including both the account number and name to assist in quality checks.

⊙ Dual-sided documents should be avoided. If a dual-sided document is used, formally designate the document as a dual-sided document and make note in the design that the document is dual-sided. That way, if the document is scanned, a reference point for the page is visible.

⊙ Documents should orient vertically rather than using a mix of vertical and horizontal for simpler readability during record review.

⊙ Documents should be 8.5 by 11-inch standard size instead of legal size or folded in any manner to reduce labor time in document handling if any of these documents need to be printed or copied.

⊙ Colored paper should be avoided because some colors don't scan clearly.

⊙ Multi-ply forms should be avoided because they will decrease productivity in the scanning process.

⊙ If you must punch holes in the document to secure it in binders that are typically used on nursing units, ensure that the holes do not block actual spaces for documentation.

⊙ No staples or adhesive should be used on the document, because staples and adhesive can interfere with scanning and processing speeds. One of the most common productivity losses in the prep and scan process occurs when an organization uses staples to connect multiple page forms which then must be removed by hand.

⊙ Each form's ID number and date of last design or reformatting version date should be present in a consistent place on the document, most commonly observed on the bottom left side of the form opposite of the demographic identification data, for a consistent scanning identification region.

⊙ Forms Input and Document Capture

Information is gathered into the legal health record in a multitude of ways. To understand the content and format of the forms and build a consistent forms database for use in the EDMS, one must recognize the different input methodologies. If you understand the method of input, then you can modify and improve the input process so that it has a positive influence on the actual output of the data that appears in the document views displayed on a computer monitor or on a printed page. Most mobile devices do not have adequate surface space to display a full-page document, so their use in healthcare to review or document on records has been limited. Tablets, as opposed to smart phones, offer more surface space and are currently being explored and used by a number of facilities as a potentially practical alternative to the use of mobile workstations or personal computers.

When scanning was introduced into healthcare as a process to electronically capture images of paper documents, the design elements and formatting became critically important to successful document capture. As electronically created documents became available from various software applications, these documents had to be captured within the EDMS for the LHR alongside of the scanned documents. These electronic documents eventually would be used to provide the content that is referred to as computer outpatient laser disk (COLD) forms, which are digitally fed into the EDMS systems today. Other options of document capture into the health record include receiving documents via fax output that are then scanned or directly imported electronically into the EDMS, or receiving electronic output from another facility via a health information exchange (HIE) or some other system integration.

In physician office settings, sending information by fax from a care provider to a referring physician is common. Integrated delivery systems that manage both physician clinics and multiple hospitals typically offer a tight relationship and infrastructure, so document interoperability and exchange of data is improved, and the volume of faxed documents decreases. Email with attachments is used infrequently in physician office settings since most electronic health record software does not have email systems that allow direct transfer of a specific clinical document to another organization. Therefore, office staff printing a document, and then faxing the document to the requesting facility is the practice norm.

During the process of documentation capture, some forms originate in an electronic environment. Supporting good forms design output standards of a form that originates in an electronic environment tends to be most challenging when the health record must be printed, as it must satisfy most instances of release of information requests that are received by an organization.

The following are various ways in which data or documents become part of the legal health record:

- ⊙ **Scanning of documents:** There are several different types of documents that can be scanned into the system:
  - ○ A document that is created or preprinted on paper and completed by hand, or a document that is printed from an electronic system and then scanned into the EDMS, such as a paper consent form that a patient signs.
  - ○ A document that is produced in an electronic environment but then printed on paper and data is entered onto it manually, and the document is eventually scanned into the EDMS. A transcribed consultation report on which additional information was handwritten and signed after the document was printed is an example of such a document.
  - ○ A document that is received in paper format via personal delivery, mail delivery, or as an email attachment and then subsequently scanned into the EDMS.
- ⊙ **Key entry:** Where an electronic template is in place online, the documenter can directly access the system and complete the data necessary on the form. The document stays online as an electronic version and is integrated into the EDMS. These templates can typically be customized to a facility and, based upon the data entry recurring, may expand to required additional documentation and tasks done.

⊙ **Faxed input:** Faxing results and other portions of paper records that the facility receives from other providers into the enterprise-wide health information system is becoming more commonplace. These documents can then be scanned or transferred electronically into the EDMS.

⊙ **Electronic to electronic interfacing:** These electronic documents make up the core of the electronic health record in an EDMS and they represent all those items that are created using electronic templates within the core HIS, EHR, or a legacy system. Legacy systems pertain to older source systems that may run on different platforms than the enterprise-wide health information system or EHR such as pathology results, medication administration order sheets, or other ancillary systems.

Based on the author's experience, approximately 60 to 80 percent of the document content in hospitals today originates electronically. This large number of electronic forms coexisting with paper documents is one of the reasons that conducting a forms inventory early in the process of preparing for an EDMS can be very helpful. The transfer process between the EHR and the EDMS must be monitored carefully through the process of electronic document reconciliation to guarantee document integrity within the LHR. Document integrity is ensuring that all documents are compiled in a timely and accurate matter within the legal health record. Any reviewer of the legal health record should be able to see a document in its entirety including any amendments, edits, authentication or signature, corrections, or alterations that are made past the point of patient discharge from the episode of care, without having to revert to previous versions of documentation. In other words, the documents must be stable and not dynamic if edited, so as to ensure document integrity.

⊙ Electronic Document Reconciliation

The final process in forms management is the act of document reconciliation. Electronic document reconciliation can refer to several distinct processes related to the use of an EDMS, each of which is discussed as follows.

COLD Reconciliation

The intent of a COLD reconciliation process is to balance document counts between the sending system, which is typically from the main HIS or EHR environment and the receiving system, which would be the EDMS. Other systems may also provide electronic content or interfaces into the EDMS, such as Health Level 7 (HL7) Admission, Discharge and Transfer messages that help to provide demographic data into the EDMS. Knowing the exact number and type of documents or messages being sent from the one system and matching that information to the information that was received in the second system encourages document integrity. The COLD reconciliation process also reduces the chance of noncompliance because of missing documentation in the electronic health record.

A complete list of the COLD feeds will be necessary for the facility to continuously track, and this list becomes part of the forms inventory discussed earlier in this chapter. Figure 6.3 shows a sample tool that can be used to track the COLD interfaces.

During this reconciliation process, the sending system creates an electronic audit log that displays the volume and type of each of the electronic messages or feeds sent to the EDMS. The EDMS should in turn provide a count of the documents received from the external systems.

Figure 6.3   A sample tool that can be used to track the COLD interfaces for reconciliation purposes if an automated report does not exist

SAMPLE COLD FEED DAILY RECONCILIATION FORM	TODAY's DATE:	INTERFACES RECONCILIATION CHECKED BY:			
NAME OF SYSTEM or SOFTWARE APPLICATION	COUNT OUTGOING FROM SYSTEM	COUNT INCOMING TO EDMS	DISCREPANCY (OUTGOING/ INCOMING)	CORRECTED?	COMMENTS
(X Vendor) Medical Transcription Reports	420	420	0		
(X Vendor) Medical Transcription Reports	320	320	0		
(X Vendor) Medication Records	640	638	2	Y	Corrected incorrect account numbers (duplicate)
NAME OF SYSTEM or SOFTWARE APPLICATION	OWNER of SYSTEM/ FORM (name/ department/ phone number)	FORM OUTPUT NAME	FORM NUMBER	Interface Completed	Sample Attached
(X Vendor) Medical Transcription Reports	Gail Archer/ Medical Transcription/ Ext 8569	History & Physical	XHP	Y	Y
(X Vendor) Medical Transcription Reports	Gail Archer/ Medical Transcription/ Ext 8569	Operative Reports	XOP	Y	Y
(X Vendor) Medication Records	Don Smith/ Pharmacy/Ext 4568	Medication Administration Records	XMAR	Y	Y

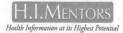
Health Information at its Highest Potential

This reconciliation process should occur daily to maintain a balance between the two electronic systems. The reconciliation process can help to quickly identify any system or report failure and avoid the issue of missing documentation or stalled interface feeds and their subsequent negative impact on patient care due to lack of complete information. The quality of your document interfacing determines the overall quality in measure of completeness within your EDMS.

Paper Document Receipt

The reconciliation of documents other than COLD feeds begins at the daily accounting for discharged patient records. In those clinical areas that still provide a paper chart of any type, the need to collect these records, identify the information that has already been captured into the EHR, and track those items that are still missing is a necessary task that should be completed daily in healthcare facilities. The paper document reconciliation process is another key factor in validating the completeness of the health record. Facilities sometimes have difficulty obtaining cooperation from clinicians to release the record for processing after the patient care episode is complete. One solution that has proven successful in some facilities is to complete an internal incident report like those that would be logged with a risk management department on any missing health records at the time of patient discharge. In this way, the incident report is used to document any missing charts or large sections of thinned records that would indicate a gap of time between the discharge of the patient and the beginning of the processing of the health record. These gaps could potentially be used to denigrate the integrity of the record content and thus tracking trends in missing or delayed records during the chart pick-up process actually encourages accountability of the clinical staff to complete their documentation on a timely basis and make the records available for pick-up immediately upon patient discharge.

Having a discharge list printed for all inpatient and outpatient discharged patients is an effective method of collecting these discharged records from each patient care area once the episodes of care are completed and the patient is discharged. Each one of these daily discharges should have a corresponding electronic and, possibly, a paper record as well. At a minimum, documentation should be present, regardless of the storage mechanism, for each and every patient encounter or episode of care. As the HIM staff collects these records, all missing charts should be identified and the charge nurse asked to authenticate that a search has been done and the record content could not be located. *Missing charts* are defined as charts missing from paper rounds collection or charts for which no electronic documents are visible within the EHR or EDMS. Identifying missing records and authenticating that a search has been done helps provide an audit trail that accounts for potential gaps in documentation and therefore mitigates risk in any circumstance where a delay or lack of knowledge concerning the whereabouts of a record within the facility occurs. Some facilities use the occurrence of a missing chart as an opportunity to complete an incident report. When missing health records are treated as a serious quality indicator, the likelihood for successfully resolving these issues is much greater.

As facilities collect the discharge records, some routinely dispose of or shred any documents that are COLD-fed, because those documents would have already been entered into the system. Other facilities keep the COLD documents with the paper records and destroy both together when they reach their retention destruction date.

◉ Best Practices and Innovation Takeaways

There are many tried and true best practices in forms management. These practices have been used for years in both healthcare and nonhealthcare settings. Historically, healthcare systems have paid close attention to excellence in forms design when the health record was primarily paper based on fear that poor data would cause poor decision making or the risk of liability.

It seems that the explosive growth of technology and automation has created a somewhat lackadaisical and chaotic approach to document management within a healthcare organization, and one that has focused more heavily on documentation input instead of output and processing. In some cases this situation has arisen due to no single party taking ownership, from an administrative perspective, for document or data integrity within the health record. In other cases, the situation has arisen simply because the root cause has been ignored and the discipline necessary to standardize design in both input and output of the legal health record has not been enforced. The result of this disorganization has:

- ◉ Increased the potential liability for facilities;
- ◉ Decreased the potential for success in interoperability of data between health information exchange and users of the documents;
- ◉ Led to potential decreased reimbursement; and
- ◉ Brought about a less than efficient workflow for employees in healthcare facilities.

Some of the best practices that can help assure effective forms management that were reviewed in this chapter include:

- ◉ Establishing a forms committee with ultimate authority and approval for all additions, deletions, and modifications to EHR or EDMS content reflected in the legal health record
- ◉ Establishing forms design standards for the organization
- ◉ Utilizing bar code identification on all documents that need to be scanned
- ◉ Using just-in-time forms wherever possible, meaning that the documents are generated as needed and not created from blank or prepopulated documents
- ◉ Centralizing control of downtime forms within healthcare facilities
- ◉ Conducting a forms inventory and maintaining an up-to-date hard copy binder of all existing form outputs for training and validation purposes

⊙ Establishing a robust electronic document reconciliation process

⊙ Establishing an accountable discharged patient health record pick-up process

Once good forms are created, using them and maintaining them efficiently and effectively (whether in paper or electronic formats) is critical to creating and maintaining a successful legal health record.

REFERENCE

FormFast. 2014. FormFast FastFlow EMR Solutions. http://www.healthitoutcomes.com/doc/formfast-fastflow-emr-solutions-0001

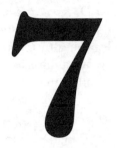

Chapter

7

Paper and Electronic Health Record Retention Issues

The primary intent of an electronic document management system (EDMS) within the electronic health record (EHR) is to provide a repository to easily access all the documents and data within the legal health record (LHR) relative to a patient stay. But, the ability to properly archive and purge these documents is equally important. Document retention guidelines and the methods used to purge and destroy electronically created or maintained documents are a topic of heavy debate, including a disagreement in the healthcare community as to whether EHRs should be destroyed at all. Many healthcare facilities are still struggling with the costs and legalities of storing, retrieving, and destroying paper medical records, complicating these retention and destruction issues further.

Hospitals have historically managed record retention quite differently from physician practices. Physician practices tend to retain records for the minimum length of time, and hospitals tend to keep records well beyond the required years of retention. Hospitals might keep records beyond retention requirements due to fear of potential litigation, increased access of older records for reference and research due to higher than average patient readmission rates, or simply because the storage space is available; the true reasons remain unclear. Regardless of the reason, archive, retention, and destruction standards remain a murky topic, without a single definitive answer to help guide the various healthcare facilities. As more hospitals have acquired medical clinics and merged their staff as well as their legal files, policy decisions around retention have become more complex and difficult.

⊙ Conducting a Legal Health Record Inventory

Multiple existing resources guide healthcare facilities through the process of creating a formal definition of the LHR, which could be considered a subset of the overall designated record set (DRS) for an organization. The definition of an LHR in one facility may be quite different from the definition at another facility, based on each individual organization's needs, state or federal laws, standards in the medical community, and the interpretation of existing guidelines and published best practices. The American Health Information Management Association has a practice brief, see Appendix E, *Fundamentals of the Legal Health Record and Designated Record Set*, which provides detailed definitions and various matrices and policy suggestions to help guide a facility through the process of defining the legal health record. The author recommends that any organization that is considering or has already started implementing EHRs have a continuously updated LHR policy and definitions in place.

It is critical to recognize that the LHR serves as the business evidentiary record for healthcare facilities, and thus the documents in the health record, by default, become the facility's LHR, whether the LHR originates or is retained on paper or in an electronic file. Therefore, as one considers applying retention and destruction guidelines to documents, healthcare providers must tackle the underlying issue of identifying the records that actually exist and their format.

As a recommended best practice, keeping an up-to-date inventory of existing records will provide the following benefits:

- Ability to identify the location and the volume of records stored in paper format
- Ability to identify the volume of activity and the amount of space required for records stored in electronic format
- Ability to identify the costs associated with storage, retention, and destruction of records
- Ability to identify the security controls necessary to protect information in the records
- Ability to identify any risk issues associated with record storage and access

The process for performing the inventory includes the following steps:

1. Review existing logs, records, and spreadsheet inventories.
2. Identify locations of the paper and electronic records.
3. Review storage areas, including offsite areas, to conduct physical inventories where possible.
4. Update or create new logs, records, and spreadsheet inventories as needed.
5. Identify record retention guidelines specific to each record type and update the record retention policy as needed.
6. Identify the records that need to be purged or destroyed and identify a mechanism to purge or destroy the records.
7. Update the inventory after destroying records.

To take a proper health record inventory, first be aware of the current location of the records. Surprisingly, knowing where the records are kept, whether in various computerized applications or a physical storage location, is more difficult than one would expect because multiple individuals may manage the various types of records and their locations. In a hospital setting, the director of health information management is typically designated as the legal custodian of records, but he or she may not know where health records are stored in other departments within the organization that generate records, even if those records are part of the LHR. In physician practices, the administrative support person, the business office manager, or even the physicians themselves may hold this role of being responsible for long-term record storage. Due to inadequate knowledge and information about historical records, one can conduct a truly robust LHR inventory only by painstakingly interviewing every manager of each department within a hospital and manually searching all locations for the presence of archived paper records. In addition, a software application inventory must be taken to identify the applications are used for long-term archive of clinical records or reports. In some cases, due to management turnover, knowledge may be lacking about what records are stored and where they are stored. In these cases, a physical review of the site via the security or plant manager may be necessary, along with interviews or inspections of existing EHRs' software configuration to determine presence of records.

The important role of the EDMS as the LHR in an electronic environment once again comes to the forefront. The EDMS provides the only way to capture, as a single encounter, a complete record within an inventory that can stand alone as an evidentiary business record, unlike the disparate pieces of data that may be retrieved within the template-style displays that are typically found in many EHRs.

Many lessons learned in the paper record maintenance environment can be applied to the electronic environments of an EDMS or an EHR, and guidelines for record retention and destruction apply to each environment, even if the standard time periods for retention may not be the same. Within each location of stored records, the following elements should be collected and included on the LHR inventory whether stored in paper format, electronically, or on alternate media such as films, cassettes, audio, logs, and other types on nonpaper media:

1. Date ranges for volumes of records, such as July 1980 through March 1995

2. Types of records, such as Inpatient, Day Surgery, Observation, Emergency, or Dr. xxx Clinic

3. Physical storage location or software system, such as HIM Department Microfiche Storage Cabinet, Basement, Building 2, Level 4, X Software System, Version 1.0, PACS system XYZ, Master Patient Index, or X System

4. Equipment noted, such as Movable File System or Open Shelf Filing Racks

5. Volume of records, such as X number of linear inches or feet, X number of boxes, X number of files, or X number of bytes

6. Manager or owner of records by area, including name and contact information

During the inventory process, certain issues will inevitably arise. Risk management and potential legal counsel should be sought for guidance in these areas, prior to any final action. Table 7.1 outlines typical findings and suggested potential remediation actions.

Table 7.1 Potential legal health record inventory discoveries and suggested remediation actions

Potential Inventory Finding	Possible Remediation Actions
Paper or electronic records that should have been purged and destroyed based on retention standards, but are still in existence.	Evaluate options for purge and destruction. At the time the records are purged and destroyed, make a permanent inventory of destroyed record ranges and update the LHR inventory.
Evidence of document integrity issues including degradation of physical containers or charts or potential inability to access electronic files within a software system.	Evaluate remediation actions that include cleaning, reorganizing, repairing, upgrading software, and backing up software.
Evidence of potential security or privacy risk, due to either lack of physical access controls or inadequate sign-on control to protected health information within active or inactive medical records in the EHR or EDMS.	Review existing policies and procedures for potential modification. Investigate and report, using proper channels like an incident report or quality committee, any discovered incidences of breached information that would create noncompliance with the Health Insurance Portability and Accountability Act (HIPAA) standards (HHS 2014).
Evidence of gaps in records or the inability to obtain complete portions of paper or electronic medical records.	Review existing policies for handling missing records. Investigate and report using proper channels like an incident report or quality committee and take remediation action as necessary. Log any identified missing records or record ranges as part of the inventory.
Outdated or noncompliant storage or software contracts.	As part of the inventory, review any existing storage, access, processing, and archiving of documents and records related to the LHR. Review any of these contracts and begin remediation processes to revise and amend contracts so they are HIPAA-compliant and support existing retention and destruction policies for the organization.
Evidence of nonstandard record processing, storage, or retention compliance policies.	Variations within a single organization can occur due to mergers and acquisitions, different time periods, different leadership interpretation, and even different policies and procedures. Best practices suggest having consistent guidelines for record storage and retention throughout an organization to simplify the process of release of information and purging and destruction. Tackle this issue by forming a team to address this situation and creating a master policy around the processing, maintenance, retention, storage, and purging of both paper and electronic data.

Once all locations have been reviewed and the inventories updated with current and accurate information about the paper or electronic records, review retention guidelines that are in place. The approved and current retention guidelines should be compared to the existing records that were discovered during the inventory process and, based on the specific retention and destruction policies in place for the institution, commence an action plan to bring records into compliance with the retention standard. The following section reviews certain archive and retention considerations for healthcare facilities.

⊙ Documentation Tales from the Front Lines

Experience teaches us what does and does not work in managing health records. EHRs and EDMSs are relatively new compared to the paper medical record management process. Learning can be easier if shared through anecdotal examples that demonstrate the type of risks encountered in systems without proper forms control or without a Level 3 EDMS application infrastructure in the LHR. The anonymously provided examples described in the following sections originated from actual incidents reported by a variety of health information management professionals as testimony to the glaring need for improved management of clinical documents in healthcare organizations. Each section starts by describing a risky documentation practice and then explains what should have happened and why the practice is dangerous, followed by what needs to happen next.

Case Study 1

A hospital has an EDMS in place that acts as the facility's LHR. The hospital also has an active forms committee. A nursing unit purchased fetal monitoring equipment and is documenting clinical results on the equipment, which does not interface with the EDMS.

What should have happened and why this is dangerous: The forms committee should have provided guidelines that prohibited the nursing unit from using the equipment unless the narrative information was interfaced into the EDMS or the information could be recorded elsewhere within the nursing documentation system. Fragmented portions of documentation can be missed during the coding workflow, resulting in recording an inaccurate diagnosis that might be inaccurately passed on for future care or release of information.

What needs to happen next: Storing alternate media such as the fetal monitor strip itself in other archiving equipment like the fetal monitoring system is acceptable as long as noted in the LHR policy. However, the results related to the actual strips—including any narrative interpretation—must be documented in the clinical system, which then should be interfaced into the EDMS for long-term archival purposes.

Case Study 2

An EHR application in a hospital allows physicians to select all unsigned items and authenticate these with a single keystroke without reviewing documentation content.

What should have happened and why this is dangerous: This practice is equivalent to having someone rubber-stamp a signature onto multiple pages, without the clinician authenticating that the contents have been reviewed and are correct. Indicating that content has been reviewed when it has not been reviewed is misleading and can heighten potential liability for a practitioner and the facility.

What needs to happen next: The sign-all feature should be disabled. While some EHR systems allow quick scrolling or opening and closing of each document in succession prior to signing, any application that does not allow the practitioner adequate time for reading, editing, correcting, and authenticating a signature is not supporting the integrity of the record.

Case Study 3

Pathology reports display a more detailed pathological diagnosis than the one listed on the discharge summary from the physician, creating inconsistency in the final LHR. At this same facility, multiple consulting physicians are often called into a single case, documenting differing diagnoses on the same patient.

What should have happened and why this is dangerous: Inconsistent documentation causes confusion in the LHR, which can impact reimbursement, lead to poor medical decisions, and decrease the quality of the outcome for the patient. In addition, inconsistent documentation can cause a delay in the patient's discharge from the facility, impacting the efficiency, costs, and effectiveness of the care. Different and conflicting diagnoses can occur; the conflicts need to be resolved by practitioners and settled by the attending physician of each case prior to patient discharge.

What needs to happen next: Guidelines and ongoing education in clinical documentation improvement should be provided to the medical staff. An interactive query process should be put in place to identify and track such variances and provide the opportunity for the clinicians to correct any discrepancies prior to the patient's final discharge.

Case Study 4

EHR functionality allows cutting and pasting from previous progress notes and history and physician documents into a patient's record if the patient is readmitted within 10 days. While allowing cutting and pasting is typically a facility's choice, some software does not contain a control to be able to turn this functionality off, therefore introducing the element of risk in the documentation.

What should have happened and why this is dangerous: While the guideline of 10 days attempts to limit a reuse of information, any incidence of cutting and pasting is not recommended due to the risk of inaccurate documentation. Carrying over old medication, resolved conditions or diagnoses, and procedures performed can be dangerous to patient care and cause fraudulent billing. Cutting and pasting sections of documentation should not be allowed in any circumstance.

What needs to happen next: The LHR should read as a chronological story that adequately addresses the history of the patient, including reference to past conditions. But, past conditions should be clearly delineated from any currently treated conditions that are using resources or being addressed in the current episode of care. Carrying over demographic information is acceptable once registration validation has occurred, and cutting and pasting should not be allowed by policy and by system application blocks.

Case Study 5

A facility purchases an EDMS but does not interface all electronic documents from other source systems, making documents such as physician orders, lab results, and cardiology results together with the scanned images inaccessible to the EDMS workflow applications. Instead, these documents are stored in the EHR, causing the HIM staff to access multiple systems for documentation review during coding, release of information, and deficiency management.

What should have happened and why this is dangerous: This type of system fragmentation leads to reduced productivity of HIM staff and presents the potential to miss capturing records for release of information. The fragmentation also increases the likelihood of LHR inconsistency and potentially decreases revenue from the coding process if fragmented results are not accessed properly. In addition, in the long term, these records cannot be archived properly and destroyed following a records retention schedule. All information should flow into the EDMS to create a single episode-based LHR.

What needs to happen next: A remediation plan should be put into place to begin interfacing existing electronic documents into the EDMS. Wherever possible, all historically fragmented records should be retroactively loaded into the EDMS to make the LHR as complete as possible.

Case Study 6

Medication orders are administered within the EHR, but without adequately identified documentation of the condition for which the medication was ordered.

What should have happened and why this is dangerous: Without a matching diagnosis, the record leaves a question in the reader's mind concerning why a particular drug was ordered. The questions can confuse coders and result in lost reimbursement and increased external record quality reviews. All medication orders should contain a matching diagnosis explaining the rationale behind providing the prescription. The same can be said for any order—if a physician orders a consultation, the reason for the consultation should be explained.

What needs to happen next: Wherever possible, electronic forms redesign should be utilized to include data entry fields that mandate adding information on diagnoses to any new medication order. Additional education can also be provided to the clinicians to explain the importance of this level of detail in their documentation to support the flow of the patient story within the health record.

Case Study 7

A physician provides advice via email to a patient. The patient does not follow the advice, but the email does not become a part of the patient record. The patient goes on to sue the physician. Had the e-mail become part of the patient record, the entire a situation could have been avoided.

What should have happened and why this is dangerous: Due to increased use of e-discovery practices that now can uncover even the tiniest discrepancy in electronic documentation, all interactions with the patient must be charted. Fragmented communication trails make omissions look like negligent care, and that situation is misleading in the story of the care of the patient.

What needs to happen next: Any communication and interaction between a practitioner and a patient, even one via electronic means such as email or telephone call, should be formally documented somewhere in the health record. That documentation must become part of the patient's LHR. Dating, timing, and receipt confirmation messages from formal system sources should be used. Personal email should not be used to communicate with patients.

Case Study 8

During the merging of two hospital systems, staff discovered that one facility had inadvertently destroyed several years of patient paper records that had not yet met the retention date.

What should have happened and why this is dangerous: Premature destruction of records can be problematic from a patient care and a release of information perspective. Destruction should have occurred only at the time the patient record actually met the retention and destruction date.

What needs to happen next: Documentation of the incident should be provided by the healthcare organization's legal representative. When requests for release of information are received for specific destroyed records, a copy of the letter stating the facts should be included with the information that is released. To alleviate these types of problems, establish an oversight committee that approves and maintains retention standards.

Many more examples could be cited that identify various points of risk within healthcare organizations related to recordkeeping. Despite this, progress should not be halted on the use of EHRs. In fact, the opposite is true—by learning from examples where risk and problems are identified in today's systems, the next generation of EHR and EDMS tools can be configured to avoid these issues. EHRs can help eliminate problems in access and storage associated with paper records. Providing adequate functionality, security and privacy controls, and nonfragmented access through use of EDMS technology can improve workflow dramatically, reduce risk, and further demonstrate the value of the EHR.

⊙ Archive, Retention, Purging, and Destruction Considerations

A facility must take into account a variety of factors when creating an LHR retention policy or determining how records are archived into various storage stages. These factors include reviewing

- ⊙ Any existing statutes of limitation within a state;
- ⊙ Federal guidelines;

- ⊙ Accreditation guidelines;
- ⊙ Payor reimbursement guidelines;
- ⊙ Medical association guidelines; and
- ⊙ Hospital association guidelines.

Other factors influence the length of time and the location and method of storing health records, and these considerations have both pros and cons associated with either shortening or lengthening the retention period based on organization preference and experience. The following sections review these considerations.

Physical Space Limitations

For facilities storing records primarily in a paper format, space and the cost of that space is a key consideration. Many facilities choose to locate paper records in a centralized area to avoid labor costs associated with retrieving the records from disparate locations. Some facilities choose to move storage offsite to further avoid using real estate that can be better utilized for direct patient care activities. Certain equipment, such as photocopiers, scanners, fax machines, computer terminals, bar code readers, printers, microfilm or microfiche readers, and other specialized equipment, may also need to be located in the file storage area. In an electronic environment, due to the need to be able to print, copy, and scan various electronic documents, the need for equipment space must still be recognized, even if the bulk of the records are stored electronically in an EHR or EDMS. See chapter 9 for a more in-depth discussion of the virtual HIM department of the future.

Staffing

Staffing considerations also can impact decisions about record retention. The heaviest use of health records at a typical facility occurs within three years of the primary episode of care. For the majority of patients, not returning to a facility within a three-year period indicates a high likelihood that the patient won't use that particular facility or provider again, and the likelihood increases with each passing year. High retrieval request rates within a facility dictate a high ratio of staffing to retrieve records. While retrieving a physical or paper record typically takes longer than retrieving any electronic file, the greater the number of records stored electronically, the longer the retention period. Furthermore, the more disparate the record content is within the system, the longer electronic record retrieval becomes, until the time to retrieve the electronic record can rival and even surpass the time needed to retrieve records within a paper environment. Follow a firm retention policy, because the budgetary implications and ripple effect that can be felt by an organization that does not adhere to a policy can be disruptive to managing file retrieval staff, particularly related to the function of release of information.

Destruction Rationale

The question facing many facilities is whether to destroy or retain the files, and when to do so. The facilities often have a difficult time answering this question.

HIM professionals should evaluate state and federal retention guidelines for specific retention requirements. Once a retention standard indicates that a record *can* be destroyed, debate often still occurs concerning whether the destruction should actually take place. Sometimes, an adequate budget for file review, purging, and destruction does not exist. At other times, individuals are afraid to permanently destroy a record just in case a request for the information occurs in the future. While an information request might occur, a facility must question the value of certain aged data. Certainly, a single case might indeed provide a clue in research or treatment, and, for this reason, many facilities across the United States adopt a policy of minimum retention standards. That is, if the records can be destroyed 10 years after the discharge encounter date, then the records will be retained for 10 years before purging begins. In some facilities, different standards of retention are applied based on whether the original record belonged to a pediatric minor—18 years or under—or an adult. This approach of selective retention and compliance to a destruction policy reduces the liability of the facility in producing historical records and provides relief from the continuously growing staffing demand in the release of information area.

The following table is an example of differing retention standards a facility may choose to apply based on the August 2011 *AHIMA Retention and Destruction Standards Practice Brief*.

Federal Requirement	State Requirement	Accreditation Requirement	AHIMA Recommendation
Hospitals: Five years. Conditions of Participation 42 CFR 482.24(b)(1)	Healthcare facilities must retain medical records for a minimum of five years beyond the date the patient was last seen or a minimum of three years beyond the date of the patient's death. Oklahoma Dept. of Health Reg. Ch. 13, Section 13.13A	Joint Commission RC.01.05.01: The hospital retains its medical records. The retention time of the original or legally reproduced medical record is determined by its use and hospital policy, in accordance with law and regulation.	Patient health and medical records (adults): 10 years after the most recent encounter.

Source: AHIMA 2011.

However, there is a disagreement over this minimum record retention policy in some of the clinical and academic research facilities, where research is done across many years of records. In other facilities, a sentiment presides that being able to produce older records may actually help to protect an organization because it can provide a particular piece of data. One thing is certain, though; no "one size fits all" model exists, so examining the balance in costs as opposed to number of requests for historical records beyond a set amount of years may help organizations set a policy. Does the staff time needed to manage these records and the obligations within release of information protocol that requires staff to review and release the years of kept records balance the desire or need of clinicians for records to use in clinical research? It can be a costly and confusing conundrum to decide which records to purge and destroy and how to purge and destroy them, but establishing a policy is important when working to evolve to a complete EHR management environment.

With rapidly changing technology, medications, and treatment protocols, the value of retaining the record, even in electronic form, needs to be questioned. Just because information exists does not mean the information will be helpful, and, in fact, the information can lead the practitioner down an erroneous path of treatment if assumptions are made from past records. Unfortunately, this situation has been exacerbated in electronic record systems, because the information is easily accessible, transferrable, and can be replicated partially or in total without considering whether partial information can be misconstrued by the receiving party. In situations where problem lists, medication lists, and allergy lists are longitudinally updated in a system but various episode of care impact those lists at other facilities, information can be incomplete, misleading, and potentially dangerous.

Within a paper record and associated with a Level 3 EDMS, information is limited to a non-dynamic record that provides a stable review of data associated only with the time period of the episode of care. This non-dynamic record eliminates the guessing component within fragmented and discrete data EHRs concerning whether the information is currently valid or historically valid, even though both appear with a template that doesn't identify the current status of the data element. With careful capture of each episode of care, a personal examination, and by updating information, a practitioner can avoid an overdependence on data in older or template-driven record sets in which there might be inaccurate data fields.

Isolation of Records and Ability to Destroy

To isolate a record means to be able to capture it wholly in its native environment to purge or destroy its content. All associated elements of the actual LHR must be captured as a single episode of care to purge it electronically or physically from its storage location. A Level 3 EDMS environment has the capability to purge records, typically by date, type, and location or facility of origin, so that only the master patient index (MPI) remains. The destruction log can then be used to track the details of the records that were purged, and in an electronic environment, the system would indicate the record has been archived. Currently, EHRs that do not isolate all documents into a permanent, archive-ready record might have a difficult time purging episode-specific data and documents as a single episode of care.

Methods of Destruction

For paper records, methods of destruction are typically more labor-intensive and costly. The LHRs inventory assists in identifying the location of records, but due to the physical bulk of the records special arrangements must be made to retrieve, remove, and destroy the records. Savings are realized after records are transitioned into an electronic environment, because the physical removal and destruction costs are no longer an issue. In addition to paying for the removal, facilities often pay an additional fee for secure destruction means, such as shredding or burning the records, since the confidential information contained within the records prohibits using regular trash disposal through paper haulers to dispose of the records. If records are stored at an outsourced storage facility, the record destruction and removal process must also be supervised and paid for by the facility that owns the records. In cases of outsource storage, destruction terms should be part of the standard contract, defining intervals of regular purging and destruction so that the healthcare provider avoids paying space storage charges for records that can be legitimately purged and destroyed. In an electronic environment, destruction involves technologically removing the complete episode of care from all systems, so that the data is no longer viewable or searchable. The data cannot simply be archived to a different software platform or system, because the ability to include the data in access and review for release of information purposes would still exist and cause a labor strain on resources and an increased liability for the organization to provide swift access and response to requests for these cases.

⊙ Best Practices and Innovation Takeaways

Paper record storage is still a considerable and costly burden for the majority of healthcare facilities who have not yet been using complete EHRs for a long enough period of time for all historical purging to take place. Of those organizations, many have chosen to bring record storage back in-house, which is considered a best practice, but others have continued to use outsourced record storage companies. Many of these companies have evolved from microfilm and microfiche processing agencies to offsite record storage houses, and today these companies may offer themselves as providers of scanning services. Regardless, knowing what guidelines should be in place before contracting with an outsource storage service is helpful. An article in *For the Record* outlined some specific tips in helping to negotiate a contract with outsource storage vendors:

1. Record storage companies should have guaranteed retrievability of at least 99 percent of the records requested within 24 hours, or there should be a refund of fees for the storage in proportion to the percentage of pulls per month.

2. Record storage companies should be asked to store the records in terminal digit order (or in whatever order the facility originally had them stored) and not placed randomly on shelves, locating them only with a bar code. This becomes a nightmare if records need to be relocated into another filing system or storage center.

3. Whenever possible, avoid box storage and ask that records be stored in open shelf storage for better and more rapid access. Urgent records should be retrieved with one-hour turnaround. Watch for extra fees for stat turnaround time and increasing fees over time.

4. Record storage companies should provide the facility with an ongoing inventory on a monthly basis, electronic and printed format, if requested, so it has an index and volume of all records stored at any time.

5. Record storage companies should provide an aging report to identify those records that should be destroyed according to retention schedules. When records are kept beyond retention life, there are often extra fees attached to the storage of those records.

6. Ensure that there are limited or no fees for returning your records if you discontinue using off-site storage.

7. Ensure that the contract for off-site storage has limitations on annual price increases and does not have a hidden auto-renewal clause.

8. Ensure that you know the hours of access should be 24/7 and that there is adequate security, fire protection, insurance, and bonded employees working in the off-site storage area.

9. Ensure that the transport vehicles moving your records are insured for damages of loss, theft, physical damage, or breach of confidentiality.

10. Ensure that you have unlimited access to the premises in order to inspect the storage conditions of your records. (Gates 2008)

In an electronic environment, the EDMS can assist a facility in easily identifying ranges of electronic records using episodes of care that can be marked for purging and then destruction, which can happen in bulk. Coordinating this destruction on an enterprise-wide basis can be difficult, so the following best practice tips should be used in handling electronic purging and destruction:

⊙ Identify the individual who is responsible for purging and destroying electronic records. This person can be determined only after completing the LHR inventory, formalizing the retention policy, and defining the LHR for the organization.

⊙ Ensure that a mechanism exists in the master patient index encounter level to visually identify the records that are purged from the system and are no longer available for viewing. This mechanism should display the actual date of purge or destruction.

⊙ If patient medical records exist outside the main EDMS or EHR environments that are considered part of the LHR, these additional records should be purged and destroyed as well.

⊙ Retain destruction logs indicating which records are no longer available.

The purge and destroy operation can be simplified by ensuring, as a best practice, that one (and only one), permanent archived electronic file exists and serves as the LHR for the facility. Therefore, regardless of any redundant electronic copies of the record that exist or of disparate pieces of data in results reporting or other software systems, an organization can successfully manage electronic archive, purge, and destruction processes.

REFERENCES

AHIMA. 2011 (August). Retention and Destruction of Health Information. Appendix C: AHIMA's Recommended Retention Standards (updated). http://library.ahima.org/xpedio/groups/public/documents/ahima/bok1_049250.hcsp?dDocName=bok1_049250

Department of Health and Human Services. 2014. The Privacy Rule. http://www.hhs.gov/ocr/privacy/hipaa/administrative/privacyrule/index.html

Gates, M.A. 2008. A tall order. *For the Record* 20(2):10. http://www.fortherecordmag.com/archives/ftr_01212008p10.shtml

Chapter

8

Technical and Organizational Challenges

An organization faces multiple challenges when it tackles the type of monumental changes that come with an electronic document management system (EDMS) or electronic health record (EHR) system. These challenges often include technical issues such as physical connectivity between sites, database integration, interface obstacles, interoperability of system data, and choosing the right equipment. The biggest non-technical challenge may be finding the vendor best suited to be a software partner. This chapter provides an overview of these issues and examples of ways organizations may overcome struggles on their journey from hybrid to fully functioning EHRs.

⊙ Multihospital Systems and Mergers

Healthcare facilities come in every size, shape, and form, yet have similar issues when attempting to evolve from a paper or electronic hybrid environment to a full EHR. Table 8.1 provides examples of some factors that may influence both the speed of this evolution and the type of systems chosen include.

In the healthcare industry today, within the 5,723 registered hospitals, facilities continue to merge, separate, create partnerships, and buy and sell off contingent care sites in an effort to remain competitive and current (AHA 2014). This restructuring activity also extends to the physician practice environment, where a number of individual and multiple group practices are joining hospital-integrated delivery systems in efforts to create economies of scale. These joint physician-hospital organizations (PHOs) provide labor efficiencies and reduce costs when purchasing equipment and supplies, educating staff, and providing care coordination. But these benefits also create new technological and operational challenges in an industry that already has great difficulty supporting change and modernizing its systems.

Table 8.1   Factors that influence the migration to a full EHR

Issue	Factor
Ownership of the facility	Religious, not-for-profit, corporate
Location of the facility	Single site, multiple sites, multiple states
Type of facilities	Hospital only, hospital-physician mix, physician only, critical access, long-term acute care, acute care, specialty, or other types of facilities
Human resources	Information technology (IT), health information management (HIM), use of outsource staff, use of consultants
Technical issues	Variety and number of disparate software systems, number of legacy systems, percentage of documentation created electronically as compared to paper-based documentation

These technical and operational challenges include lack of interoperability of data and document exchange between systems and differing sets of policies and procedures guiding the production, processing, and retention of patient records.

Software systems designed to support complex care systems can cost hundreds of millions of dollars for larger facilities. These robust systems may be unaffordable at smaller facilities that rely on partnering with larger organizations to support their information technology needs. The return on investment of the EHR is difficult to measure because of its large scope and impact across many processes and departmental operations. As leadership at these healthcare facilities make decisions concerning the best ways to invest capital dollars for software applications related to the EHR, consideration should include the cost of the software, implementation or build initiatives, cost of initial and ongoing staff, as well as clinician training, ongoing upgrades, integration, and maintenance of these systems.

As facilities merge, each facility's staff brings expertise in their current operational expectations and processes, but the merged facility is faced with the challenge of either simultaneously maintaining multiple systems or selecting one of the solutions and retraining the staff and clinicians. In the end, the merged facility faces the task of essentially installing a new system for the site whose software is being replaced, which can be a great benefit or a serious disadvantage to a facility merger, depending on the position in the tool selection process and whether a change will be beneficial. Undergoing software replacement can take several years to accomplish and as a result, these organizations tend to accept and maintain less than optimal functional applications once they are implemented, rather than initiating the work and the cost of replacing a flawed system. The decision to change or replace a system can also be mired in cultural debate and frustration, since users of these software components in various departments are very loyal to their system and their system's vendor. These users have integrated specific changes in their workflow around a system's particular configuration and therefore do not easily embrace change and the retraining needed to adapt to a new system.

Certain systems are considered legacy systems in that they may be maintained despite the implementation of a replacement application. These types of systems generally contain a large volume of patient-specific data, but due to technical constraints or cost constraints, data from the legacy system is not converted into the replacement system, so the legacy system must be retained to provide access to that data. The maintenance of both a new system and a legacy system creates another degree of hybrid record fragmentation that must be considered as an EDMS is implemented. Policies should be created to describe the ongoing maintenance of the legacy system, including how long to retain the documents or data in the system and to address ownership and access issues for any information that may be retrieved from the system. Retention should meet state and federal regulations (refer to the discussion in chapter 7). If located outside of the health information management (HIM) department, one must also consider who can access the legacy system to retrieve records for the release of information function.

When facilities merge, they should create a transition team to oversee the merger. Systems interoperability or compatibility should be a key consideration when making decisions about the software the newly formed partnership will retain. Consider the following factors when making decisions about software relative to an EDMS or an EHR:

- ◉ Is an enterprise-wide master patient index system in place that provides cross-referencing against each individual facility medical record number? To create a single unit number use across each facility, one must be able to reference legacy numbers to identify older volumes of retained paper records as well as any existing electronic health records in the legacy system. A good practice for healthcare organizations to engage in is a systemwide clean-up across all master patient indices before merging any data that then can provide a clean start in the database for any upcoming system implementation, including that of an EHR or EDMS.

- ◉ Is there an existing EDMS in place that is being used at any of the facilities as the LHR? If so, this existing EDMS could be a leading factor in deciding how to create a path for all facilities to fully adopt a successful electronic health record management (EHRM) program.

- ◉ Merging systems of data has associated costs. Prior to merging, all existing data should be backed up. This backup helps the facility maintain the ability to retrieve data both visually and in print. Pricing quotes from vendors for merging may include costs for both the originating system database and the receiving system database. The significant lead time needed to prepare for and then merge data should not be underestimated.

Regardless of the final decisions made in merging systems that contain health records; policies and procedures will also need to be updated to reflect jointly agreed-upon and legally approved definitions of the LHR, and every effort should be made to incorporate any source or legacy system documents and data within the EDMS.

As facilities grow in size and number of entities, management of these records becomes quite complex and labor intensive. Consider managing the health information function from a centralized regional perspective relative to EHRs processing. Current trends in centralization have allowed facilities to move to effectively manage electronic documents and other records through a centralized model of support, utilizing outposts known as virtual HIM departments at satellite facilities. See chapter 9 for more details about virtual HIM departments.

⊙ Software Integration Issues

Software integration issues for EDMS can be challenging from a technical and organizational perspective due to the large quantity and diversity of data and reports created in the myriad of source systems that comprise the core of the EHR. The software systems may have completely different underlying programming languages and platforms, making interoperability of data a challenge. Some systems may be configured to operate within a web-based or cloud environment, and others require desktop software components. Since private and personal health information is contained within the records in these systems, the degree of protection offered to the records may be of consideration when transferring or moving data. Some of this data may need to be available to remote workers, and other information may need to be integrated with external systems like workman's compensation claims systems and social security databases. The need to integrate with external systems makes the use of firewalls, passwords, encryption, and other secure data methods an additional consideration when setting up an EDMS or EHR.

Within the EDMS, as previously discussed in chapter 6, all forms, documents, and reports used as part of the patient's care must be included as a part of the legal health record. These documents, whether scanned into the system or received through electronic interfaces into the EDMS, must be reconciled and linked with the appropriate episode of care via the account or encounter number originating from the MPI. The documents may be received via Health Level 7 (HL7) automated messages or may be received directly from the originating or source systems. Documents typically may be received as .pdf files, .rtf files, or html-formatted files. All must then be converted into viewable document files within the EDMS system that become part of the chronological electronic legal health record.

In the case of HIM-specific software applications that support the workflow within an EDMS, additional software integration and automation must be evaluated and occur to successfully implement these systems. Most commonly, the core systems discussed in the following sections involve the greatest degree of integration needed within the EDMS.

Incomplete Record Processing

Health records, electronic or paper, are analyzed for deficiencies. Whether this occurs at the point of scanning or at a later point in time, the file needs to be integrated with the chart completion system. This integration allows clinicians to complete documentation within an episode of care as an addendum process. In some instances, the chart completion system is embedded as a part of the EDMS. In other cases, it may reside within another software application, making integration or interfacing a necessity. Clinicians must have the ability to add a signature for document validation and authentication; clinicians also need to be able to enter additional information into the patient record via either dictation, structured, or unstructured data entry. These entries must all be signed, dated, and timed in accordance with applicable state rules and regulations or Medicare Conditions of Participation. Systems may be able to create the signature, timing, and date automatically as a byproduct of clinician secure access into the completion system.

The physician order entry system presents another aspect of incomplete record integration. As an order for an element of care occurs, it should correspond with an expected receipt of a document or a report. For example, if a consultation is ordered by a neurologist for a patient, a corresponding neurology consultation report should be documented, typically within 24 hours of the order. If a lab or radiology test is ordered, a corresponding document containing these reports should be received. Within the deficiency or incomplete system, an automatic flag could be set to identify if that specific document related to the fulfillment of that specific order is either present or missing, which equates to a chart deficiency for either the report or the signature.

As a correlation to the completeness of the record from an order-fulfillment perspective, the transcription and dictation process also needs to be integrated with the EDMS to support the workflow of deficiency management. Consider the situation in which a clinician dictates a report such as a history and physical. Once that history and physical document is integrated into the EDMS from the transcription system, an automatic flag would appear to the clinician the next time he or she signed onto the system, notifying the clinician of the need to read and authenticate that document. Thus, when updates occur to any transcribed documents, the link between the transcription system and the deficiency management system is active and reflects the current status of the document, its completion status, and notifies the clinician of any needed review and authentication. When the HIM analysts finish final incomplete record processing, they can then validate any final documents needing completion or authentication within the system with the aid of the integrated transcription and deficiency management systems within the workflow component of the EDMS. Monitoring the record during the active patient care process, as opposed to waiting until post-discharge identification, will result in a more complete and accurate patient health record and can assist in improving overall record processing turnaround times, decreasing chart delinquencies for incomplete record processing.

Coding and Abstracting

Coding and abstracting of data workflow functions were discussed thoroughly in chapter 3, but the software integration requirements are also key to efficient processes. Coding and abstracting requires access to encoding and grouping software, requiring multiple types of interfacing between separate coding and abstracting functions, the charge description master, the master patient index functions, and other applications that support the coding process. The output from the coding and abstracting functions must be able to flow directly into any post-discharge editing or bill-scrubbing software, electronic data interfaces for outgoing claims processing, and any facility decision support databases. Data from these type of applications is relayed into claims and billing systems, including claims clearinghouses, to produce the Uniform Bill 04 (UB04) and Centers for Medicare and Medicaid 1500 (CMS 1500) data fields necessary to submit for reimbursement from third-party payers. Each facility may have a unique mix of applications that touch the data between the time that the data originates in the coding and abstracting systems until the data appears on the final bill.

As computer-assisted coding (CAC) and clinical documentation improvement (CDI) software applications are introduced into the enterprise's information technology environment, the receipt and organization of the specific document files becomes even more important. Users of CAC and CDI technologies are finding the time-savings benefit is related to better access and workflow of the documents since this improved access and workflow had been missing in their previous EHR-only environment. When working from the base of a well-implemented EDMS solution, the adoption of advanced technologies such as CAC and CDI applications, layered on top of the EDMS software, provides even greater potential for more efficient workflow in the coding and abstracting functions for the HIM department.

Any software that contains coding or coding-related data requires a degree of integration and maintenance of various code sets and edit tables. These tables can become time-sensitive and content-sensitive. Code sets and edit tables sets are changed at various times throughout the year, and if any of the systems becomes out of sync due to a delayed update of edits or coder content tables, that system may generate an error or inappropriately flag a problem with the coding-to-billing workflow. Use a master chart or table to identify each of the components, the owner of the component's maintenance, and scheduled dates for updating tables as a control for the ongoing successful integration of these system components.

Release of Information

In the release of information (ROI) function, any ROI software application needs to be integrated with the MPI episode-specific data and allow access to the source system containing original or historical records, including any legacy systems. This integration is needed to validate requests and allow staff to retrieve records to fulfill a request for release of patient health information.

Ideally, the ROI system will also integrate into two additional systems: a back-end billing or accounts receivable system and an external portal for reviewing records. The billing system interface may be used to invoice those who make release of information queries for the cost of the reproduction and delivery or mailing of the reproduction copies of the record. Fees for this service are defined by facility policy and guided by state law reimbursement guidelines in the department of public health codes if present.

The external reviewing portals, if utilized by a healthcare facility, can provide another access point for patients, clinicians, or other requestors for electronic records, thus reducing distribution and delivery costs. If portals are used for direct self-serve access to health records, the facility must consider how to display integrated records stored on different media and you must establish policies that clearly delineate what will and will not be available to requestors via the portal.

⊙ Technical Standards and EDMS Component Technologies

No single technical standard exists for healthcare software related to electronic document management systems or the EHRs system. However, understanding the common usage and elements involved with the configuration of the EDMS is important for any facility considering use of the EDMS as its legal health record and as a critical component of its EHR strategies.

The following grayed sections were authored and updated by Deborah Kohn, MPH, RHIA, FACHE, CPHIMS, principal of Dak Systems Consulting for the 2011 book *Enterprise Content Management and the Electronic Health Record*, by Sandra Nunn, MA, RHIA, CHP.

Since the late 1980s, when one of the technologies of electronic document management systems (EDMSs), document imaging technology (also known as document capture technology), first was implemented in US healthcare provider organizations to manage (namely, digitize) the organizations' massive amounts of medical, financial, and administrative analog documents, many health information management (HIM), healthcare information technology, and other related professionals did not understand that document capture technology is not the *only* technology of an EDMS.

Automatic Identification Technologies

EDMS technologies allow documents to be automatically identified. The following are examples of EDMS automatic identification technologies.

Automatic/Intelligent Document Recognition

Automatic/intelligent document recognition (ADR/IDR) recognizes the layout and content of generic form types. In healthcare organization EDMSs, ADR/IDR is used to recognize digital and analog form categories.

Bar codes

Bar codes are machine-readable representations of data, typically dark ink on a light background to create high and low reflectance which is converted to 1s and 0s. Originally, bar codes stored data in the widths and spaces of printed parallel lines. Today, bar codes also store data in patterns of dots, concentric circles, and text codes hidden within images. Bar codes are read by optical scanners or scanned from an image by special software. In HIM department

EDMSs, bar codes are used to eliminate the manual indexing of document type, patient name, provider name, and medical record number, and such, as well as medical record separator sheets during the digital scanning process.

Intelligent Character Recognition

Intelligent character recognition (ICR) allows different styles of hand printing and handwriting to be learned by a computer. Most ICR software includes a self-learning engine (namely, a neural network) that automatically updates the recognition database for new handwriting patterns. In healthcare organization EDMSs, ICR is used to recognize documents' hand-printed or handwritten numbers or abbreviations on analog orders, in analog progress notes, and such (Nunn 2011).

Other experts dealing with ICR have stated,

> the industry average for intelligent character recognition (ICR) is about 70 percent. That means that 3 out of every 10 characters are read incorrectly or aren't recognized with a high enough confidence to be considered accurate. One should never expect 100 percent accuracy in any forms processing project, but a successful ICR application should exceed 70 percent accuracy. Accuracy of 90 percent or higher is considered good, although that's still 10 bad characters out of every 100 (Scanlan 2013).

Optical Character Recognition

Optical character recognition (OCR) is the electronic translation of analog typewritten or printed text into machine-editable text. Early OCR systems required system training to read specific typed or printed fonts. Today, OCR has a high degree of recognition accuracy for all fonts. Some systems are capable of reproducing formatted output that closely approximates the original scanned page including images, columns, and other non-textual components. In healthcare organization EDMSs, OCR is used primarily to recognize the printed text on claim forms.

Optical Mark Recognition

Optical mark recognition (OMR or mark sense) is the process of capturing data by requiring a page image to have high contrast and an easily recognizable shape. Mark sense is distinguished from OCR by the fact that a recognition engine is not required. That is, the marks on a page are constructed in such a way that there is little chance of not reading the marks correctly. One of the most familiar applications of optical mark recognition is the use of #2 pencils on paper-based, multiple choice-type question examinations. In healthcare organization EDMSs, mark sense often is used for physician office analog super bills and charge tickets.

Enterprise Report Management (ERM) Technology

Enterprise Report Management (ERM) or computer output to laser disk (COLD) are EDMS technologies that store computer output to—and indexes computer output on—digital storage media. Once stored, the computer output can be easily retrieved, viewed, printed, or distributed. Today, computer output consists primarily of batch-generated computer reports with data that are report formatted. Electronic health record (EHR) batch-generated computer reports include EHR system bills or invoices and management reports. (*Note:* Any system external to the EDMS, including the core EHR or HIS within an organization, can provide electronic output from any report formatted template or system into the EDMS in order to be included in the legal health record.)

Document Management (DM) Technologies

The following are examples of EDMS document management (DM) technologies that control and organize documents.

Document Assembly

Document assembly allows documents to be automatically retrieved in the correct order, based on predefined, user-specific rules and tables.

Document Version Control

Document version control allows documents to be automatically assigned version numbers. For example, this includes daily laboratory test result reports (version 1) vs. cumulative summary laboratory test result reports (version 2); preliminary radiology procedure result reports, unsigned (version 1) vs. final radiology procedure result reports, signed (version 2); transcribed operative reports (versions 1, 2) vs. signed transcribed operative reports (version 3) vs. amended transcribed operative reports (version 4). Typically, only the most recent or last document version is accessible for view purposes.

Document Check-in/Check-out

Document check-in/check-out allows users to collaboratively review and edit shared documents without concern about who might be simultaneously updating the document and to view all the entries made to the shared document. Clinical teams who author electronic progress notes is an example of this important document management technology.

Document Security

Document security consists of all the technical document tools to protect, control, and monitor document access (for example, unique user identification and authentication, audit trails, automatic log-offs, and biometric identifiers) to prevent unauthorized access to documents transmitted over a network.

Document Imaging (Capture) Technology

Document imaging technology is the EDMS technology that captures (via scanning, faxing, or automatic identification technologies), stores, and retrieves documents—regardless of original format. Contrary to popular thinking, document imaging (capture) technology is one component technology of an EDMS. Because HIM departments have worked with massive amounts of analog medical record document for so many decades, currently HIM departments use this EDMS component technology more than they use the other EDMS component technologies. As such, too often this EDMS component technology is synonymously and incorrectly used to describe an EDMS. When all internal and external medical record forms, notes, letters, reports, and messages are generated, stored, and distributed electronically, the use of this EDMS component technology will be drastically reduced and all the other EDMS component technologies will be used more frequently.

Forms Processing Technology

Forms processing—an EDMS technology that electronically delivers paper forms for printing and completion, accepts scanned paper forms and extracts data from the boxes and lines on the forms to populate databases, and utilizes eForm templates that look like paper forms for online data entry and data collection. Forms processing is also known as electronic forms management or automated forms technology within EHR environments. Since patient medical records consist of hundreds of forms, even with EHRs this EDMS component technology is important for healthcare organizations.

Workflow or Business Process Management (BPM) Technology

Workflow or business process management (BPM) technology in an EDMS (or any other type of information system) technology is the most important component technology in an EDMS (or other information system). BPM technology automates business processes, in whole or in part. EDMS workflow and BPM technology passes documents, information, or tasks from one user to another for action according to a set of business rules (Nunn 2011).

⊙ Architecture and Requirements

Several key architecture concepts or principles must be analyzed as healthcare provider organizations move forward with an EDMS. These concepts and principles include:

- A service-oriented design allowing applications to be broken into services that can be accessed by other applications and systems. This approach creates powerful composite applications based on the functionality available in applications across the enterprise.

- Event-driven tools to capture key changes in business needs. These changes can then be used to effect instantaneous changes to processes and workflows and the underlying systems that support them.

- An alignment with life-cycle support processes and workflows that account for the collection, dissemination, and use of the information to help organizations make better decisions.

- High levels of application scalability, performance, and reliability.

- An ability to leverage existing technology investments to minimize unnecessary technology and to provide maximum benefit.

In addition, the architecture must support key requirements including support for:

- Patient-related clinical, administrative, and financial documents and processes and workflows

- Nonpatient-related administrative documents and processes and workflows

- A healthcare organization's existing technology environment and agreed-upon standards

- Ease of maintenance with minimum customization

- HIPAA security and access standards

- Centralized and distributed components, such as point-of-service (point-of-care) capture

- Retrieval of patient-related documents between and among healthcare facilities

- Open standards

Document Capture Hardware

Today's major document capture hardware vendors offer well over 100 products from which to choose, with devices for analog document scanning, analog photographic film scanning, fax, and multifunction (scan, print, copy, fax). Each product depends on the business use case(s) articulated by the healthcare organization. Analog document scanning use cases include but are not limited to capturing:

- Analog hard cards (for example, plastic), such as insurance cards, driver's licenses, and identification cards as well as biometric readers (for example, fingerprint) in patient registration or other front-end processing areas

- Externally generated analog documents that enter the organization by a patient (or representative), postal mail, courier, or fax in point-of-service or other appropriate processing areas

- Analog documents in either a centralized or decentralized and distributed mode in back-end processing areas
- Analog documents that are determined to be either current or historical, active (namely, frequently retrieved) or inactive (namely, infrequently retrieved), or combinations (for example, historical-active) in appropriate processing areas
- Analog documents in a production mode (via the organization's network) or mobile mode

Today, document capture hardware ranges from under $300 to over $80,000 per unit and includes the following, general features:

- Monochrome versus color, with resolution at 300 dots per inch (dpi) letter/portrait and 200 dpi letter/portrait, respectively
- Speeds from 8 pages per minute (ppm) to 130 ppm
- Automatic document feeders (ADFs) from 10 to 500 sheets of paper
- Software for the Mac, Windows, Android, and iOS operating systems
- Daily volumes from 100 to unlimited number of scans (Kohn 2014)

⊙ Document Capture Software

EDMS software in a healthcare environment typically encompasses both document workflow software and document capture software. When selecting a software vendor, evaluating the quality of the document workflow component should be the focus based on how well the EDMS software supports the functions described in chapters 2 and 3.

Hundreds of technical specifications apply to an EDMS's document capture technology software. The following are sample technical specifications that should be included in a healthcare organization's request for proposal or similar EDMS document capture technology acquisition approach.

The technology recognizes whether the captured (namely, scanned) document is a single or double-sided form.

The technology recognizes that if a form is single or double-sided but the single or double-side is blank, the blank single or double-side can be automatically deleted.

The technology automatically rotates and saves a document to its correct view position (for example, 90 degrees) based on the position of the identification code on each document.

The technology includes an electronic whiteout or redaction feature to reduce the amount of blank, scanned document storage.

The technology supports the capture of a variety of data types and files, including but not limited to document image data and files, ASCII data and files, word processing text data and files, HTML data and files, JPG files, and computer output files.

The technology allows document types to be global or similar category. In other words, the same version of a global document type, such as an advance directive or driver's license, can be retrieved for all episodes of care until such version needs updating or replacing.

The technology provides the capability to later capture documents and appropriately insert the documents to an already established patient episode-of-care record or employee file.

The technology operates without its own document image index database. In other words, the technology image enables the organization's existing data repositories that have their own database management systems for record searches.

The technology interfaces with a healthcare organization's master patient index (MPI) or other primary indexing module for the receipt of all or selected index data.

The healthcare organization's MPI updates or other primary indexing module's updates come through the interface to automatically update the document index database.

The technology captures and stores the existing number of index keys in the EDMS's index database, so that searches can be made using a number of index keys.

The technology's database management system allows the healthcare user to retrieve records by the patient's current, active and unique medical record number, as well as by any previous, inactive medical record number(s). (Kohn 2014)

⊙ Other EDMS Hardware Considerations for the HIM Department

In addition to the large document management devices, individual desktop scanners are used by the EHR and EDMS applications in an organization. Most notably, these small and relatively inexpensive devices are seen at the patient access or registration point in a facility so that they can scan identification and insurance care information and external documents. Desktop scanners are a helpful addition to the typical HIM employee workstation; they can be used to scan a document received separately from the main batch of records, such as late or loose reports, or to capture incoming mail requests for release of information. Individual scanners are also ideal for use in the quality review process to recapture a document that may not have been captured clearly. In any case, individual scanners can save time and avoid backlog waits for the use of a single scanner in a work area.

Bar code scanning devices are another type of hardware used in the processing of analog documents and as a tool to expedite various workflow processes within the EDMS. Bar code scanners can be hand-held style, similar to the wands used at a retail store for scanning product bar codes; and used to capture, for example, a list of location names or physician names that an employee would need to access to retrieve the correct case or workflow path.

Stationary barcode reader devices can also be used and would work best when checking in volumes of records that contain an external bar code on the outside of a folder. The bar code can be moved beneath the stationary reader device to register the item and record its movement. Stationary barcode readers can be particularly helpful in tracking the movement of an existing historical paper health record if it is retrieved for release of information or review upon readmission of a patient into a hospital, particularly if the patient's chart has not been converted electronically yet.

Computer monitors are an important hardware component of EDMS systems because the record images are viewed through these devices. As an industry standard, EDMS users work with dual, side-by-side monitors to best utilize the software applications. This setup is particularly important because users can display a large resolution view of electronically input or scanned documents that may contain handwritten information display on one monitor, and the input operations—whether coding, deficiency management, MPI searching, or other workflow application—on the other monitor. Lightweight liquid crystal display (LCD) monitors come with adjustable stands, touch screens, and a myriad of other functionalities.

Using an appropriate mix of document scanners, monitors, printers, barcode readers, and software provides an ideal environment for the records management functions within the HIM department.

As architectural requirements change over time, certain core technical standards need to be considered within the EHR and EDMS. Advancement in these technologies will continue to blur the lines between traditional EHR environments and the advanced workflow functionality present in EDMS applications. As facilities experiment with combinations within these two platforms, the division in source content of the record will become less noticeable to the end user, and therefore a more efficient way to display content of the patient record during the patient's episode of care, while maintaining the infrastructure and integrity of the LHR.

Regardless of its hardware components and technologies, the EDMS should be a vital part of the organization's strategies to deliver a complete, compliant, current, consistent, and concise way to manage all clinical documentation that becomes the organization's business and legal health record.

⊙ Selecting an EHR/EDMS Vendor Partner

Selecting an EHR/EDMS vendor partner is perhaps the single most important decision in the process. HIM leadership participation in this decision, as the custodian of the legal health records, and the person responsible for information governance of the workflow involving that record, is critical prior to selecting an EHR or EDMS software vendor as a trusted partner and developing a request for proposal (RFP). Multiple factors should be reviewed. The following sample questions provide insight into top 10 important considerations.

☑ Does the vendor involve appropriate health information management leadership involved in pre-sale presentations to the facility or is the system being marketed and proposed only through information technology, clinical leadership, or other department of the organization?

☑ Does the vendor have an AHIMA certified staff member or independent HIM consultant available to be involved in system configuration and implementation?

☑ Has the vendor offered a visit to the site of a similar healthcare provider to view live functionality of the proposed solution?

☑ Do both the EHR vendor and the EDMS vendor support using the EDMS as the foundation for the LHR?

☑ Has the vendor been able to demonstrate the solution's capability to integrate all existing clinical documentation from any source system into the EDMS?

☑ Does the vendor solution have the ability to provide role-based protective access to comply with privacy regulations and the need-to-know philosophy to protect patient privacy?

☑ Does the vendor solution have complete workflow functionality that can integrate with the facility MPI?

☑ Can the vendor solution demonstrate that document input views are consistent with document output views upon printing of any form, report, or document that is defined as part of the LHR and designated record set?

☑ Can the vendor solution demonstrate that the complete legal health record for a single episode of care can be permanently purged?

☑ Are audit trails available for all access, change, printing, and destruction of data—across all timed versions of documentation?

Each facility should define those factors that are most important to the purchase decision in question. The amount of budget, the stakeholders involved with the decision, the number and types of facilities are involved in having to obtain the equipment are all factors that should be taken into consideration during the equipment selection process.

⊙ Best Practices and Innovation Takeaways

As a best practice, healthcare facilities are beginning to more tightly integrate the EDMS and other system applications that are involved in the creation of documents and reports that will become part of the LHR. Service-oriented architecture (SOA) is a popular term being used to describe a number of information technology network configuration and usage designs that assist in accomplishing the goal of improved integration for end users. SOA has been described by Microsoft as "not just an architecture of services seen from a technology perspective, but the policies, practices, and frameworks by which we ensure the right services are provided and consumed" (Sprott and Wilkes 2014):

Sprott and Wilkes go on to discuss three characteristics of SOA:

⊙ *There is real synchronization between the business and IT implementation perspective.* For many years, business people haven't really understood the IT architecture. With well-designed services, we can radically improve communications with the business, and indeed move beyond alignment and seriously consider convergence of business and IT processes.

⊙ *A well-formed service provides a unit of management that relates to business usage.* Enforced separation of the service provision provides us with a basis for understanding the life-cycle costs of a service and how it is used in the business.

⊙ *When the service is abstracted from the implementation, it is possible to consider various alternative options for delivery and collaboration models.* No one expects that, at any stage in the foreseeable future, core enterprise applications will be acquired purely by assembling services from multiple sources. However it is entirely realistic to assume that certain services will be acquired from external sources because it is more appropriate to acquire them. (Sprott and Wilkes 2014)

When SOA is used in healthcare relative to an EHR or EDMS application, understanding the concept of the collaborative relationship between EHRs and EDMSs and the characteristics presented here will make addressing the needs of healthcare providers an easier task. Although the EDMS is the foundation and centralized document capture and storage area for the legal health record, its workflow applications touch many other aspects of the patient care and revenue cycle, as well as many other system applications. To provide a seamless, service-oriented architecture means that the applications and documents in the EDMS can be used for business process tasks such as chart completion and retrieval of historical records, and also be accessed by another portal or system applications that need to integrate with the EDMS. Therefore, the end user—whether a physician, patient, or health information staff member—can all view a consistent document that is presented through the EDMS, but that appears as if an alternate software application is presenting it, providing the user with a particularly seamless experience. As state-of-the-art EDMS applications advance and discrete data and document images can interplay in an easier fashion, defining the workflow processes and application in each business application will drive the use of the appropriate system to clearly document the story of the EHR encounter.

Part of synchronization is controlling versioning in documents. This is key document management technology for an EDMS that differentiates it from other template-based systems. Since the EDMS continually receives dynamic electronic reports fed from the core EHR, the document integrity can only be maintained if the change information is visible to the end user.

For example, a preliminary radiology procedure result report may be an unsigned document internally identified as Version 1; while a final radiology report, authenticated and displaying a physician signature is identified as

Version 2. The same situation is true for operative reports, other diagnostic tests, transcribed reports, amended reports, or documents that require co-signatures such as reports dictated by medical interns that may require countersignature by an attending physician after a note is entered into the system. Typically, only the most recent or last document version is accessible for viewing to an external user, but more sophisticated EDMS systems are beginning to display multiple layers and levels of report versioning to more easily visualize the life cycle of a particular document. Use of natural language processing as an adjunct to the EDMS also assists in identifying certain documents and their intended sequence, and can assist in displaying these versions in the appropriate order as required by various end users.

Another example of how an EDMS provides excellence in version control would be in a situation where an allergy to a certain drug is reported by a patient upon admission into a facility. The physician may make a treatment decision based on that information and prescribe a different medication to treat the condition, but it was ineffective resulting in a bad outcome. In reality, subsequent to being treated, the patient reported that they did not provide accurate information regarding allergies. The nurse changes the information in the EHR's discrete data database so that now the clinical record in the EHR does not display in the current report template upon which the physician acted, based on previously recorded information from a prior episode. Each medication should be documented as current, only within the episode of care in which the drug was administered. If a Level 3 EDMS does not exist, there is a risk of the longitudinal record in the EHR inaccurately displaying all medications which have been historically given as if they were provided during the current episode. If this record were to go to litigation, this would indeed cause an issue for the physician and the organization if the situation could not be explained. However, this situation would be avoided and easily explainable in a court of law with the appropriate use of an EDMS, displaying all changes as visible addendums on the record after document completion. This, in turn, mitigates risk to the facility.

Another aspect of best practice version control occurs when documents are received from external facilities. The receiving organization must identify these documents as external records for reference, yet these records are often used as the source of care and may even contain additional noted information based on the current episode of care that is entered by someone other than the original authoring clinician. Once utilized in care, these documents are typically retained as part of the existing episode of care. If external documents are received from another facility but not utilized in care, they are often returned to the original facility or provider. Having a policy in place to address receipt of external records is important because the labor involved with processing external records into the existing record can become costly. Corrections or amendments that are required on the original record must be completed only at the source facility level and not on the distributed or reference copy provided to the requesting organization for continuity of care.

REFERENCES

American Hospital Association. 2014 (January 2). Fast Facts on US Hospitals. http://www.aha.org/research/rc/stat-studies/fast-facts.shtml

Kohn, D. 2014. E-mail communication to the author.

Nunn, S. 2012. *Enterprise Content Management and the Electronic Health Record*. Chicago: AHIMA.

Scanlan, R. 2013 (July 1). Improving ICR accuracy with better form design. *ECM Connection*. http://www.ecmconnection.com/doc/improving-icr-accuracy-with-better-form-design-0001

Sprott, D. and L. Wilkes. 2014 (April 3). Understanding Service-Oriented Architecture. http://msdn.microsoft.com/en-us/library/aa480021.aspx

Chapter 9

Path to the Future through Innovation and Best Practice

Most projects begin with an idea about doing something better or improving a situation. The journey to electronic health records (EHRs) is paved with pitfalls and surprises but can also be filled with a joyous excitement. Use of electronic document management system (EDMS) technologies can make the journey less perilous if organizations and providers understand lessons learned from past implementations. Chapters 1 through 8 have provided the rationale behind why a Level 3 EDMS is a vital component of any EHR and how the combination of forms, document management, and advanced workflow software can be used to improve efficiencies within the healthcare organization as a whole and specifically for many health information processes.

This chapter further describes the preparation necessary for implementing an EDMS as part of the EHR strategy. This chapter also provides a peek into the world of the virtual HIM department, which is one type of organizational model that can be implemented for the health information management (HIM) staff to support a successful transition from paper to hybrid to a fully electronic legal health record.

⊙ Implementation Preparation

Chapter 8 contained a detailed discussion of technical and nontechnical factors that assist an organization in selecting the vendor, software, and hardware products best suited to the workflow environment. Once these selections have been made and adequate funds have been earmarked for the EDMS project, the implementation preparation and the real work begin. At this time, an implementation plan should be developed with the stakeholder steering committee and plan. This planning process should be initiated a minimum of 12 to 18 months prior to the desired implementation go-live date. This allows for appropriate time to complete all tasks.

Figure 9.1 displays a recommendation for structure of implementation planning by its document imaging taskforce.

The following activities should be included in implementation planning, and the importance of each task is explained. Tasks are listed in the order in which they should be completed. The results in one task might be used to provide critical information needed before beginning the next task.

Forms Inventory and Legal Health Inventory

Chapter 6 and 7 describe forms inventory and legal health inventory, respectively, in detail. These chapters also provide instructions as to how to conduct these inventories, and describe the benefits in completing these inventories prior to beginning the EDMS implementation process. Organizations that skipped these

Figure 9.1   Project plan processes for structuring implementation

1. Initiating processes (authorizing the project)
   a. Contract execution
   b. Acquisition
2. Planning processes (defining objectives and the course of action to attain the objectives required of the project)
   a. Defining and documenting the scope of the project
   b. Developing the project plan
   c. Assigning the project team
3. Executing process (carrying out the project plan)
   a. Training
   b. Data collection
   c. Workflow analysis
   d. Hardware installation
   e. Software installation
   f. System configuration
   g. Testing
   h. Activation preparation
   i. Activation
4. Controlling process (monitoring and measuring progress to identify variances from the plan)
   a. Quality reviews
   b. Status meetings
   c. Overhead activities (reporting)
5. Closing process (formalizing acceptance of the project and bringing it to an end)
   a. Transition to support organization
   b. Project closure

Source: AHIMA 2003.

tasks might now have issues with out-of-control forms, redundant form names and numbers, or a lack of control over paper and electronic records—all of which are important from a maintenance, organization, archive, and retention perspective. Organizations should perform these tasks, even if an EHR or EDMS has already been implemented. As part of the forms inventory and in preparation for implementation, a full electronic document inventory must also be completed. This will identify integration requirements necessary to feed these documents into the EDMS. Both the EDMS vendor and EHR vendor containing the original documentation need to be involved and clearly understand the intended integration.

By establishing an accurate forms inventory—with proper controls in place for approval and use of ongoing documents within the health record—and maintaining an up-to-date legal health inventory, the scope of the entire HIM process and EDMS is clearly documented, understood, and can be optimized as part of the clinical care and revenue cycle in a health system.

Workflow Planning

To realize the true benefits of the EDMS software, the organization must understand, in detail, the current workflow and the proposed future state workflow.

Workflow planning includes the following elements:

- Patient type mapping
- Work queue strategies
- Software mapping

Patient Type Mapping

Patient type mapping requires flowcharting of each type of documentation or health record created. This includes information from prescheduling to discharge, relative to the movement and workflow of the patient health record. In an acute-care hospital setting, this documentation typically includes record types for inpatient, outpatient, series or recurring, emergency, and outpatients in a bed, which includes such services as day surgery or observation patients. Some patient-type categories may represent a more granular categorization of services such as newborn, obstetrical, surgical, and other types of care related to very specific units and departments within a facility. Organizations such as physician clinics, home healthcare, skilled nursing facilities, or other specialty care organizations will have their own patient-type visits that require mapping. For each patient type or category, the map should include who entered the documentation, the system into which it was entered, and how the documents are transferred until final integration into the EDMS. That way, anyone who looks at the map can easily understand the movement of a record type throughout the organization. The map will include information from point of creation to final billing. In addition, it will include whether the documentation related to the specific category of record is paper, hybrid, or electronic based.

Work Queue Strategies

An important functionality of a Level 3 EDMS implementation is the ability to utilize sophisticated workflows to queue assigned work to various workgroups. To optimize the queue functionality and its positive impact on workflow, the HIM department can set up queues for the deficiency analysis process. This process includes routing electronic records for processing to the discharge analysts using certain groupings of discharged patients or types of providers in oldest outstanding order.

Another queue example is based on total discharged not final billed (DNFB) cases that are outstanding, oldest records, length of stay, or even by payor type. A final queue is release of information work that might be automatically routed in queues for work distribution by incoming requests and sorted by legal, commercial, or patient requests based on how urgently the requestor needs the information.

In addition, automatically identifying records post-coding process can help to identify defined record sets and route them to standing review queues. For example, adverse effects of medications may be routed based on ICD diagnosis code to a pharmacy review queue. Day outliers—patients that have a significantly longer length of stay in a hospital—may get routed to a utilization review coordinator. As more sophisticated data is available and combined with the use of abstracted and zero-charge statistics and linked with the EDMS episode of care, quality reviews, core indicator tracking, clinical documentation query response trends, and complication or mortality reviews can become increasingly automated. More sophisticated and advanced workflows are developing within next generation EDMS applications and can provide increased future optimization of the system.

Software Mapping

Superimposed onto the patient type mapping, software mapping will be diagrammed to illustrate which software applications or work processes may be utilized on various documents. A second goal of this dual mapping is to identify the point within the workflow and life cycle of the EHR these software applications or work processes may be utilized. For example, birth certificate software may be used to create a birth certificate when a baby is born and generate a copy of the birth certificate that might be included in the legal health record within the EDMS. Also, cancer registry software may be used to identify and retrieve electronic records from the EDMS based on follow-up needed for certain oncology patients. It is through this process that the HIM department can provide a check and balance to ensure that no individual piece of documentation or any form is missed within the legal health record (LHR).

 Due to patient-type naming conventions and different workflow software applications, each facility will have a very unique set of maps that can be used to demonstrate changes that need to occur in current operations once the EDMS is put into practice.

Role Change and Staffing Evaluation

The adoption of an EDMS will undoubtedly change the job descriptions and productivity standards of many of the HIM staff. These human resource changes were described in chapters 2 and 3 and may require rewritten job descriptions, additional training, and even updated pay scales since, in many cases, a higher skill level and more complex decision making may be involved in job performance.

Orientation and training on new job tasks and even new skill training may be needed by staff whose roles have been modified or are brand new.

If any of the staff are union members, these types of changes and any positions that are eliminated as a result of the new technology will need to be managed through the union representative. Dealing with the union can take considerable time, depending on the relationship between the union shop and the organization.

Physical Reconfiguration

Depending on whether work processes and staffing become centralized or decentralized at the time of EDMS implementation, potential remodeling and a change in workstations may be required. Additional computer monitors will be required—two per staff member who use the system for coding, analysis, or release of information purposes—along with personal desktop scanners. As a result, desk space may need to be enlarged to accommodate these monitors and scanners. In addition, build a space for active file storage into the design that will accommodate up to 90 days of discharged records and floor room to accommodate central printers or high-speed scanners, copiers, or other bulk equipment. These records will be maintained until a final quality check can be performed, and the paper records should be destroyed via shredding or incineration once they are complete and finalized in the EDMS. Also, plan for a cart storage area, because various carts will still be used for transporting records to various workstations as the records are received from patient care areas and move through the post-discharge processing areas within the HIM department. If the plan calls for a centralized work area, and historical paper files are merged together in this space, adequate access, lighting, security, and movable or stationary shelf files must be acquired. Shelving systems may be repurposed from existing storage areas that no longer need as much space as files become digitized.

Policies and Procedures

New policies and procedures must be created or existing ones modified to reflect changes in processing when using an EDMS as a vital component of the EHR. If an LHR and designated record set have not yet been defined, create these documents during the pre-implementation phase for the system. Any alternate media or items excluded from the LHR-related definitions should also be clearly identified in these documents so that no doubt exists concerning what will be released in the request for information process. Review or create all organizational policies relative to privacy and access of the record, documentation creation, and forms management; and documentation dissemination, retention, and destruction need to be reviewed or created.

Training

Various training methods have proven successful for facilities who have implemented EDMS applications. A list should be developed for all internal and external system users to identify the level of training actually needed. HIM staff who will be working daily with the system need the most intense level of training and, most likely, larger facilities should plan to designate a dedicated system coordinator and trainer.

Clinicians may need a general system orientation and more detailed training on specific tasks related directly to them, such as document validation review and authentication. A just-in-time training philosophy should be used for this training rather than holding large training groups. The ideal time to initiate this training is when a clinician sits down to use the system for the first time.

A train-the-trainer approach can be very effective in working with small groups of individuals. Computer-assisted learning modules consisting of short-length videos or slide shows displaying entry screens may be additional helpful tools for practitioners. Using pre- and post-education tests to score familiarity with and knowledge of the system will serve as proof of adequate learning and provide users with self-confidence in using new functionality.

⊙ Time for the Go-Live

Immediately before the system goes live, you must consider a variety of issues such as productivity, staffing, setting of performance indicators, measures of success, and implementing controls to prevent deterioration of system effectiveness.

At the beginning of an EDMS implementation, productivity might take a slight decline due to the adoption of new processes and backlogs of remaining work such as handling what previously may have been paper or hybrid paper–electronic records. The facility may wish to budget for some temporary additional staff or overtime hours to assure that turnaround-time goals can be met. The learning curve is generally brief, however, and if the pre-implementation work is done properly and completely, overall efficiency will increase in the HIM processing area post-discharge, allowing for much faster turnaround time throughout all stages in the workflow than was experienced pre-EDMS implementation.

Measuring productivity is a key performance indicator in any organization. A baseline measurement should exist at the start of the project, and then be remeasured periodically for consistency and to identify any improvement opportunities. The HIM department using an EDMS should be collecting the following indicators at a minimum on a per-hour basis to set standards for staff measurement:

- ⊙ Prepping productivity: number of inches received of paper records to process
- ⊙ Scanning productivity: number of pages (two-sided pages count as two)
- ⊙ Quality checking: number of images reviewed, including both scanned and electronically received feeds
- ⊙ Deficiency management: number of health records processed
- ⊙ Coding: number of health records coded and abstracted
- ⊙ Release of information: number of requests processed
- ⊙ Loose report: number of documents processed

During the go-live, and potentially as a long-term strategy, using contract labor and staffing must be considered for those facilities that are unable to recruit and hire adequately skilled workers in the volumes necessary to support the needs of the facility. The benefits of using this type of labor, particularly in the prepping and scanning areas, are the specialized staff that might function at a higher productivity level due to their experience. An outsource company might provide the ability to provide more staff or less staff, depending on workload volume variations and an outsource company might be able to fill staffing shifts on weekends or evenings that a provider might not be able to cover adequately. Some of the contract labor companies also might supply equipment for functions such as high-speed or specialty scanning; the equipment needed to perform these functions might be more expensive than the facility can afford. The downside of using an outsource company might include the higher cost of contract labor, potential inconsistency, or incompatibility of personnel with the culture of the organization. Further, contract labor staff, unlike in-house resources, would be unfamiliar with the particular documentation styles of individual clinicians.

Reconciliation should be performed to assure that 100 percent of discharged patient records are processed and received within the system on a daily basis. This can be used as a check and balance for the facility to ensure that no paper patient charts were lost or interfaces failed and prevented electronic transfer of records into the EDMS. Table 9.1 displays an example of a tool used to collect daily scanning productivity.

Table 9.1 Productivity matrix for scanning

Week of: 11/16/2008												
Date:	11/16/2014		11/17/2014		11/18/2014		11/19/2014		11/20/2014		11/21/2014	
Scan Tech Name	Images	Time	Images	Time	Images	Time	Images	Time	Images	Time	Images	Time
					302	2						
											333	2
					176	1						
			2028	20	1480	13	1008	11	4110	40	1033	7
											456	10
			4148	45	3685	34	4111	45	1756	18	3589	37
											16910	166
			3514	39	4584	33			3210	29	1156	8
									12488	105	10072	83
			16157	213	28847	369	28555	319	20845	233		
			1803	21	4233	31	4796	38	3277	25		

Printed with Permission from Original Work for H.I.Mentors, LLC

Management practices to monitor employee performance for those individuals using the EDMS must equally emphasize data quality, document and process integrity, and productivity tracking. Methods to monitor the work output may include setting performance outcome measures such as evaluating the quality of scanned or received images. By monitoring the image quality continuously and identifying and fixing any problems such as redundant, blank, or blurry images as they are discovered, document quality can be maintained in the LHR. When building individual quality standards for staff, quality and quantity job output performance expectations must be defined for all positions.

The last consideration at the time of go-live concerns the go-live team. The team should be prepared to be available to assist with the implementation and serve as a front-line resource for users during the first week of a conversion. This team must be expert users of the EDMS and respond to any last minute questions, problems, or unexpected conversion issues. The go-live team members need to be available for any one-on-one training refreshers, particularly with the clinicians who will need assistance when first using the system, especially if the new system significantly differs from previous documentation completion systems. Due to being able to easily work with and understand the chart completion process, most facilities experience a significant decrease in the number of outstanding delinquent records, well below the thresholds required from any accrediting agency within six months of go-live. Observations show delinquent rates dropping from 50 to 60 percent to 10 to 20 percent of discharged records. Automatic controls should be put in place to ensure the signing of any verbal orders prior to the clinician being allowed to document further, which will reduce the number of nonauthenticated documents that are outstanding as deficiencies in the patient record.

Once the EDMS go-live is complete, the facility must remain vigilant to ensure that bad document and record management habits do not appear and jeopardize the success of the project. To that end, the following activities will assist an organization in avoiding problems from creeping into the EHR environment after system go-live.

1. Monitor any delayed receipt of discharged patient records from direct patient care areas in the organization. It is too easy to make exceptions in beginning to process paper and electronic records if these records are held for clinician completion and not released to the HIM department for processing. Documentation best practice is to complete documentation concurrently at the time of or immediately following a patient care encounter. Delays in completing documentation can cause clinicians to forget important information resulting in documentation gaps and in poor data integrity in the chart. Other issues that can create a poor-quality discharged record with inadequate documentation may occur due to late dictation habits, delayed review and authentication of orders and reports, cut and paste abuse, and overall lack of accountability for timely record completion. Encourage complete, concise health record charting concurrently throughout the patient care process for optimal document quality.

2. Work to prevent ongoing errors and duplicate or erroneous numbers in the master patient index, patient status changes, and other data related to the episodes of care. Errors like these can cause record content inconsistencies and tracking difficulties around the movement and processing of the record. Delays in obtaining records may cause patient care delivery errors as well as negatively impact reimbursement. Avoid exception management of problems and focus on preventing future incidents of poor data management.

3. Promptly report and attempt to resolve variations in daily reconciliation of electronic computer output laser disk (COLD) feeds from source systems into the EHR to avoid any documentation integrity problems.

4. Ensure that the forms committee continues to actively meet and review and approve any modifications, deletions, or additions to paper or electronic forms and that both the forms inventory and the legal health record are kept up to date with changes to any form.

5. Continue to maintain and actively archive, purge, and destroy paper and electronic legal health records and maintain destruction logs.

6. As further technological developments continue in the world of EHR, the facility may deploy review portals for clinicians, patients, and external reviewers. The use of health information exchanges and other data reporting sophistication will also impact organizations and demand that system integration is completed so that it avoids jeopardizing legal health record reliability within the EDMS and maintains the integrity of telling the clinical story of the patient.

The successes of the team should be celebrated. By tracking performance indicators, report cards can be developed to demonstrate improvement in turnaround time and processing efficiencies. An effective and fully functional Level 3 EDMS can result in long-term staff savings far beyond what most EHR environments alone can provide, and the Level 3 EDMS can be implemented with complete staff and clinician satisfaction concerning the workflow functionality.

⊙ The Virtual HIM Department

The virtual HIM department is a concept that has been explored and interpreted slightly differently from organization to organization. To some, the virtual HIM is the holy grail of health information management infrastructure because it is based on the theory of maintaining a minimal presence of health information staff and provides for a just-in-time approach to processing EHR. Certain functions in patient healthcare require hands-on service, such as bedside nursing care, blood draws, and physical or other therapies that depend on direct interaction with the patient. When the health record was strictly in paper format, or even in hybrid paper-electronic format, staff of the HIM department was almost always onsite at a facility and optimally near the physicians who had to provide the bulk of the record documentation. In today's electronic environment, ongoing evolution is occurring and the majority of functions performed by the health information management staff can be conducted remotely.

When the electronic record can be reviewed completely online, most of the work can be done remotely, including analysis, coding, transcription, cancer registry, purging of files, and most release of information processes. Work that requires an HIM physical presence includes

- ⊙ Management of any historical file and retrieval functions where paper records still exist;

- ⊙ Chart pick-up for remaining paper record components;

- ⊙ Urgent release of information and dissemination of printed copies of records for requestors;

- ⊙ Some clinical documentation improvement activities where interaction with practitioners is needed; and,

- ⊙ Any management functions that require onsite interaction and participation.

So how does this virtual environment evolve into reality? For multi-facility organizations or integrated delivery networks, the first action often taken is to centralize HIM functions in one location, either on a physical campus of a facility or offsite within a relatively close distance from the care system or offices. In those organizations with a true virtual HIM department, the only physical presence left in the original organization may be a small satellite office where release of information requestors can be greeted or individuals can pick up and, if applicable, pay for copies of records that have previously been requested and not been collected. One of the more difficult adjustments to make is by the HIM manager, who may have never supervised centralized or remote work teams. Figures 9.2 and 9.3 discuss considerations when setting up a virtual team's remote workers in the AHIMA Journal story, "Virtual HIM: Considering the transition to remote departments."

Figure 9.2   Considerations for setting up remote staff

Equipment and Office Setup for Remote Staff
- What furniture and equipment will the employee be expected to provide? What will the facility provide?
- Will the employee be financially responsible for the damage, loss, or theft of any facility-provided equipment or furniture?
- Will the facility provide any assistance to the employee to help set up a home office?
- Will the facility inspect the home office to ensure it meets security requirements?
- How will any facility equipment or furniture be retrieved upon termination of an employee?

Note: If the function is outsourced, the supplies and equipment are provided at the expense of the vendor.

Internet access

- Who will pay for Internet access—employee or facility?
- Will the facility determine the Internet access provider for the employee or let employees choose their own providers?
- How will access to patient information systems be handled: virtual private network, separate server for remote access, web server? (Note: these questions also apply to any work performed by a vendor.)
- What security technologies will be employed for the remote access worker? (Note: this question also applies to any work performed by a vendor.)

Computer support

- Will the employee or the facility be responsible for providing computer support?
- How will upgrades be handled? New software installations?
- For a vendor, what interfaces are needed?

References, resources, and continuing education

- Will the provider continue to purchase reference materials for employees?
- If references are provided, will they be collected upon termination of the employee?
- Will continuing education be the responsibility of the employee or facility?

Pay rates

- Will there be a different pay grade for at-home workers? If so, will the rate be based on hours or productivity?
- Will flex-time be allowed? Split shifts?
- How will attendance or productivity be monitored?

Union issues

- Will contracts require renegotiation?
- Will the union accept a different pay rate for remote workers?
- Does the union view provided equipment or furniture as an additional benefit requiring equity with other workers?

Note: if functions are outsourced to a vendor, union issues must be discussed, because the vendor may not fall under the union's jurisdiction.

Communication

- How will remote colleagues communicate with managers or receive facility communications?
- How will remote colleagues stay involved with the facility?

Source: Servais 2009.

Figure 9.3 Interdepartmental issues impacting remote staff

Requests for records
- How will requests for paper records be handled?
- Will requests for electronic records be answered by asking the requestor to view records online, printing the electronic documents, or creating a CD?
- Who will control the printing process for electronic records? Will printing be centralized or decentralized?
- What security precautions will be taken if electronic records are printed for requestors? Will the paper copies be checked out so that they can be checked in on return?

Communications
- How will remote workers communicate with physicians, patient accounting staff, and other departments when needed?
- How will other department staff communicate with remote HIM staff? How will general communications be transmitted?
- How will remote staff remain part of the facility culture? Will social events be planned on a regular basis? How will team spirit be maintained?

Source: Servais 2009.

Whether the organization decides to adopt a centralized or virtual HIM department model or a combination of both, give careful thought to the timelines, cost of change, and the subjective impact the change has on the workforce and operations. The EDMS software has increasing incremental benefits with ongoing use and efficiencies that become apparent over time.

⊙ Best Practices in Utilizing EDMS Technology

Best practices case studies show the win-win that can be experienced with implementation of Level 3 EDMS technologies. When an organization recognizes that investment in EHR software alone, without EDMS as a component, cannot result in the expected efficiencies and integrity of documentation processes, the organization seeks other solutions to obtain the needed return on investment. Going back to basics leads to the key discovery that best practice is based on infrastructure support for advanced workflow processes. This support can be found in underlying software functionality that provides for the type of labor and supply efficiencies expected with any electronic documentation process. An EDMS provides workflow satisfaction to both clinical users and HIM staff who share the responsibility for the integrity of the health record.

A brief review of key best practice principles for EDMS management follows.

1. Incorporate 100 percent of all paper and electronically created documents within the EDMS.
2. Utilize and define the EDMS as the legal health record.

3. Ensure same-day turnaround time from patient discharge to completion of any scanning and receipt of COLD documents.

4. Incorporate complete episode-of-care records available for viewing seven days per week.

5. Keep a current and accurate forms inventory, legal health record definition, and a records retention policy in place.

6. Enforce a need-to-know privacy and security policy for all users of patient-protected information and records as opposed to permitting open access. Limiting clinician documentation entry only to those practitioners who are associated with a specific patient within the system is a preferred approach. Employing a break-the-ceiling methodology by using emergency override to access a record outside those parameters will create control and audit trails for maintaining privacy compliance standards for the organization.

7. Provide a single workflow view of historical records for providers to complete any record deficiencies, including a method for secure bidirectional electronic signature authentication.

8. Archive and purge records according to a retention schedule.

9. Develop performance metrics and key productivity and quality indicators to measure successful adoption and use of the system on a continuous basis.

The need for data repositories and longitudinal data for use in granular results reporting comparisons and trends will continue to exist in the EHR systems of today and the future. Advanced technologies such as natural language scanning will use the discrete data elements available in today's EHRs to support needs of big data more easily. However, in reality, an EDMS is a vital component of the EHR and critical to a healthcare facility's success by meeting the needs of users to receive, access, manage, print, archive, and purge electronic legal health record data.

Multiple vendors exist who have been providing Level 3 EDMS solutions for healthcare for numerous years. While the EDMS core technology is stable and mature, these systems continue to evolve. The functionality of the workflow application supporting the systems also continues to advance to meet today's more complex need of document and records management in healthcare. The ability to identify more discrete data within the document images in an EDMS—even those that are captured via scanning as opposed to being interfaced electronically—is occurring today. In addition, as a result of implementing service-oriented architecture, users are seeing better integration between various software applications related to the EHR. Using innovative tools such as powerful cross-indexing processes to support cached data retrieval into appropriate work queues for a variety of needs is just one more example of technology advancements providing sophisticated functionality for end users.

Organizations that are selecting vendors need to distinguish between providers of fully robust EDMS software as opposed to providers who offer an adjunct document scanning ability. The robust or Level 3 EDMS solution contains advanced workflow software as a part of the application, including integrated functions for deficiency management, coding and abstracting integration, and release of information functionality.

When used in tandem, EDMS and EHR integrated systems assist with information identification through use of tools such as natural language processing, which, when applied, makes data access more clear. Reduction in time for clinical research trial scanning is a good example. Clinical research trial scanning has historically required reading through a large volume of health records manually to identify a very small and specific population. This process now can be completed with electronic tools, especially for first-pass screening. The ability to identify patients that can potentially receive a clinical trial for a specific type of cancer may occur more rapidly and have a positive impact on the long-term prognosis and survivability.

In conclusion, several excellent case studies and articles can be referred to as various examples of adoption of Level 3 EDMS functionality within healthcare facilities.

Evolution in HIM Operations: A Hypothetical Case Study

Health information management is a challenging profession. Unlike most healthcare professions that focus upon a single specialty or task, the typical HIM department is commonly responsible for a diverse group of functions such as release of information, record processing, coding, cancer registry, transcription, clinical documentation management, decision support, and a variety of other functions. These positions often need to be staffed by a certified HIM professional with specialized certifications and training in order to perform these functions.

During the past ten plus years, managing HIM operations became even more challenging as healthcare facilities began to shift from all paper-based medical records to hybrid environments to finally all digital records, some of which are still in a hybrid state due to the fragmentation of the documentation across various information systems. The traditional workflow functions had to be adjusted to accommodate new equipment, processes, legislative regulations, documentation methods, and expectations for improved productivity.

Rapid Changes Lead to Poor System Acceptance and Functionality Issues

Instead of an environment where the HIM director, as custodian of the medical record, provided the guidelines, processes, and physical guardianship of the paper record, information technologists and other clinicians were involved in systems selection and choosing or designing documentation input tools. These decisions were often made by individuals who did not have appropriate HIM education, certification, or training in HIM processes, and the decisions made to select a certain vendor or system tool with which to manage the EHR were often looked back upon as a poor choice as electronic records became increasingly difficult to handle.

Physicians and other clinicians quickly became dissatisfied as the current systems tended to automate dysfunctional processes in place rather than attempting to drive efficiencies based on sound workflow principles of document management. The HIM directors felt they were not involved with the decisions and were not given the chance to provide input on decisions. Other managers made diligent attempts to remain involved, only to skip being a participant in decision making around the EHR. Only a few HIM leaders, through sheer persistence, were able to become part of the EHR decision-making community and were thus able to positively influence EHR-related system and workflow process decisions.

Planning for the Future

As EHR systems began to evolve, some HIM departments were able to see the need for EDMSs in order to house the complete electronic LHR. Those that saw this need and were able to garner the support of an executive champion within their organization ensured that a Level 3 EDMS software platform was in place to support the LHR. Those that did not continued to see deterioration of data and documentation quality, increases in amount of pages per record when attempting to print the record for release of information purposes, dissatisfaction by clinicians when attempting to complete deficiencies on the record, and a general loss of being able to tell the story chronologically of each unique patient episode of care.

For those hospitals or physician practices that understood HIM workflow and recognized that eventual implosion of processes would occur without an adequate EDMS in place, the journey to a total EHR environment could begin. For those who continued to fragment the records between a system for scanned documents and one for discrete data elements that was dynamic and template driven—frustration levels continued to increase.

Planning for the EDMS Implementation

In order for an HIM department to plan for implementation of a Level 3 EDMS, they must also identify current-state as opposed to future-state operations under an EDMS environment. This can best be demonstrated in table 9.2.

A New Environment—Centralized, Virtual and Information Governance Driven

The best practice HIM department of the future is based on leadership driving toward a more solid foundation of practice principles through information governance. Information governance allows the HIM department manager to provide enterprise-wide guidance through policies for access; privacy protection; data and document processing; and usage, decision support, compliance, archive, retention, and destruction of health records.

With the adoption of a Level 3 EDMS as a strategic component of the EHR, healthcare facilities cease the debate around record management in the EHR. Instead, they begin to focus on HIM practice efficiencies, and effective management of the workflow and structure of the LHR housed within the EDMS. With all documentation now able to be accessed through a single environment, use of a virtual and centralized HIM department model can be maintained. The morale of the HIM department staff improves due to the ability to perform work functions unencumbered and with speed that allows support of the revenue cycle and access goals of the facility. Economies of scale can be adopted where multiple facilities are supported by a single centralized HIM infrastructure and expenses and supplies costs decrease.

Table 9.2   With and without an EDMS

EHR WITH A LEVEL 3 EDMS	EHR WITHOUT A LEVEL 3 EDMS
All documents and report-formatted templates containing documentation output are viewable as the LHR within the EDMS to help tell the story of the patient episode of care	Documentation may be fragmented and it is difficult to read, print, manage, archive, and purge individual or groups of episodes of care within the EHR
All major HIM workflow processes, such as record processing, coding and abstracting, release of information, and other related tasks, are supported by the EDMS so as to provide full functionality and efficiencies to the HIM staff	Individual documents may be scanned, with some rudimentary worklists and release tracking functionality, but building upon the system for advanced functionality such as computer-assisted coding or HIE interoperability becomes increasingly difficult
The foundation for improved compliance and quality clinical documentation is in place by planning for an EDMS implementation by conducting both a forms and LHR inventory and setting into place processes which emphasize standardization, consistency, efficiency, and timeliness of processing	Document and data integrity suffers with increasing errors experienced within the electronic record. More time is taken to track and resolve errors by the HIM department. Eventual staffing increases will become necessary
Ensuring complete, clear, and current documentation in a stable environment which provides stand-alone documentation for each episode of care, mitigates risk and improves compliance throughout the organization	Poorly formatted output of printed forms may occur due to use of a discrete data longitudinal and dynamic record as is found in most EHR systems. While this type of system is helpful in displaying data trends and analyzing records across a period of time, the greater the stability of the record and the software's ability to track and display revisions in the documentation, the greater the documentation integrity becomes
A higher level of physician satisfaction with the simplicity of the documentation completion and review, creating a win-win situation for all professionals responsible for documenting or managing the medical record	As clinicians are dissatisfied with workflow processes within the EHR due to anything that appears duplicative, inconsequential, or creates more work without a benefit, resistance to future system changes and lack of cooperation is likely to occur

As the staff is cross-trained, outsource functions such as record storage, coding resource assistance, and release of information can be greatly reduced, thus saving additional costs. Backlogs decrease, records get completed in a timely manner, reimbursement is optimized, and the risk of poor documentation decreases. Healthier record documentation supports improved patient care through better documentation.

By helping HIM students today understand how to manage both paper and hybrid records, and to lead the transition necessary through the Level 3 EDMS and the overall EHR through effective and detailed information governance, this evolution can be successfully accomplished.

The role of the custodian of the physical record is replaced by a new HIM leadership role to support the data and documentation integrity of the LHR as well as to protect the privacy and use of the content of the EHR. This can primarily be accomplished through a Level 3 EDMS.

Three other case studies provided through McKesson, Inc., ChartMaxx—A Division of Quest Diagnostics, and Streamline Health Inc. can be found in Appendix F. These case studies further demonstrate the powerful testimonials and successful stories of using an EDMS as the repository for the LHR and as a key component of the EHR to assist in workflow improvement. In chapter 10, frequently asked questions (FAQs) will be provided to assist organizations in their journey toward a more functional electronic record management environment through use of EDMS technologies.

REFERENCES

American Health Information Management Association. 2003. Practice Brief: Electronic document management as a component of the electronic health record, Appendix G.

McLendon, K., HIXperts. Printed with Permission from Original Work for H.I.Mentors, LLC.

Servais. 2009 (March). Virtual HIM: Considering the transition to remote departments. *Journal of AHIMA* 80(3): 38-42.

Grzybowski, D. 2008 (May). Storage solution: A plan for paper in the transition to electronic document management. *Journal of AHIMA* 79(5): 44-47.

Frequently Asked Questions

10

In the course of adopting any technology or in changing traditionally held beliefs that have to evolve to meet an unanswered workflow problem, certain questions arise repeatedly. The intent of this chapter is to provide answers to some of the common questions that are asked when evaluating legal health record (LHR) strategies that incorporate using an electronic document management system (EDMS) as part of the electronic health record (EHR) environment. These questions are based on actual questions received from clinicians, information technologists, hospital administrators, revenue cycle specialists, and health information management (HIM) professionals.

Why have many hospitals underinvested in EDMS technology if it is such a critical part of EHR strategy for healthcare organizations?

First, EDMS technology is one of the best kept secrets related to EHRs, because its operations and benefits have been poorly understood or misinterpreted as a scanning solution by most individuals except those who have hands-on experience working in an HIM department that actively uses EDMS software.

Second, EHR system vendors have not concentrated on solutions that accommodate the discharge-based episodic medical record. Most development design efforts, as well as sales efforts, have focused on handling clinician documentation *entry* during the active portion of patient care as opposed to handling the record post patient discharge and the required workflow applications necessary to support those functions.

Finally, the focus has been on the input of information, rather than the retrieval— both review and printing—of documentation that is part of the legal health record.

The retrospective access and dissemination information used as a part of the deficiency analysis, coding and abstracting, and the release of information process has often been overlooked in the overall EHR strategy, primarily due to the lack of involvement of health information management staff in the decision-making processes during the selection of EHR component software solutions.

Why have the Meaningful Use standards not addressed the use of EDMS as a required technology?

Some of the language in the expectations of the Meaningful Use standards, such as access to requests for release of information within a specified period of time post discharge, alludes to the need for a system to provide rapid access to a single episode of care. But, the language does not go to the point of listing a specific type of technology since none of the Meaningful Use standards actually define the technology.

The dissatisfaction with the current EHR-alone solutions in the market became evident after the rapid deployment and proliferation of EHR software and the recognition by the overall clinical and health information communities that generic EHRs did not contain adequate EDMS workflow process support. The dissatisfaction became increasingly evident as polls began to be published in the past few years showing discontent with the current EHR-alone solutions in the market that had been installed to try to meet Meaningful Use standards. Hopefully, future stages of Meaningful Use will contain improved standards mandating single episode-of-care document management to maintain the electronic legal health record using a methodology that mandates a stable documentation management system requirement so that the LHR is supported more robustly at the episode-of-care level. The Meaningful Use standards are also recommended to mandate electronic records which can be archived, maintained, and can be completely and efficiently purged from the system in accordance with retention standards.

Will EHRs alone ever be able to duplicate the functionality within an EDMS?

Technology is advancing at a rapid pace, and with the advancement of service-oriented architecture (SOA) solutions being deployed by organizations, better interoperability of data allows seamless viewing of various software graphical user interfaces (GUIs) between and within different vendor applications so that end users can benefit from functionality within both the EHR and EDMS solutions. These combinations of software application solutions are already becoming a reality at some facilities.

For an EHR to duplicate the functionality within an EDMS, the EHR must contain two distinct core documentation and storage components. The first piece of functionality in the software must provide for capture of discrete data elements as part of the documentation that can build longitudinal dynamic reports—reports that combine data from many individual episodes of care and update each time new information is added to the record—through templates.

The storage component must allow capture of all electronic and paper scanned documents as the complete legal health record by providing all output and reports used within an episode of care in viewable, stable, episodic and chronologic document folders.

This combination of technologies, which are represented dually by the EHR and EDMS today, can accomplish both of these functions. Wrapped around a layer of workflow business process management tools, this combination of technologies has the potential to achieve a fully functional EHR environment.

In chapter 6, the importance of forms inventories and legal health record inventories as the first step toward creating the legal health record and a necessary step prior to implementing an EHR or an EDMS is emphasized. Why have so few organizations appeared to have tackled this important task?

As excitement rose in the industry in the move from paper to hybrid to electronic document and records management in healthcare, the historical paper records seemed to take a back seat to the forward-looking EHR development. Since the function of managing the paper records often occurred in a back office, basement, or even offsite remote storage facility, this function (along with release of information of the content of these records) was not as evident due to the number of other competing interests that vie for investment dollars for the decision makers who have the duty of selecting EHR solutions. In addition, with the newness of automation in patient records, and the historically limited information available on EDMS use in healthcare, many of the decision makers would not have realized the importance and criticality of the post discharge and documentation workflow needs, and therefore the benefits of a Level 3 EDMS to a successful electronic environment for recordkeeping.

For some organizations, the task of creating and maintaining these inventories is not only viewed as a non–patient- or non–physician-centric, low-priority task, but creating and maintaining these inventories is extremely difficult even if the support is available. The task is time consuming, involves all departments, and may have to rely on external consulting expertise to be conducted properly. Keeping these inventories up to date also requires a commitment to data and document integrity and the ongoing leadership of a stakeholder-driven forms committee. Without an executive champion who recognizes the value in these activities in the long run, the investment in these important controls can be missed.

What is likely to occur in the long run if a facility ignores the need for an EDMS system and insists on trying to use a discrete data system as its legal health record instead of the EDMS?

Evidence already exists of the problems that arise just by reviewing recent literature, which is full of news reports of clinician, executive, and HIM professional dissatisfaction. As an example, in October 2013 HCPro (now Fortis) published findings from an EHR benchmark survey in which more than 60 percent of HIM professionals responded that both data integrity and privacy/security of the medical record has either stayed the same or gotten worse with their EHR implementation (HCPro 2013). Other problems can be predicted and are already appearing in some facilities.

Increase in staffing is needed for HIM functions such as coding and release of information (ROI). The increased staffing results from the coders having difficulty in reading through the record in a clear format. Release of information staff may experience problems accessing and printing the record in response to requests for ROI, especially in facilities that have not continued to permanently purge and destroy the electronic records. In other cases, multiple errors and problems in documentation can cause an increase in positions that handle data integrity and audit functions. An EDMS would typically resolve these issues by making these workflow processes more efficient.

With the growth of health information exchanges and large-scale big data use, interoperability of data and forms standardization become more important due to the need to transfer documents between facilities. Transferring documents has proven increasingly challenging without an adequate forms inventory or workflow infrastructure to manage the complete legal health record. An EDMS would typically resolve these issues by providing improved checks and balances, by monitoring forms, and by managing data errors and corrections in a controlled environment.

As the legal community becomes educated and more aware of the flaws in the EHR-only model of documentation, including the discrepancies present in systems that do not capture a stable document image and instead are displaying templates that dynamically change each time to reflect the current state in time the data is accessed, litigation activity will undoubtedly increase, with potential loss of revenue for providers who have not addressed this concern.

What is the recommended remediation plan if a facility has not implemented a Level 3 EDMS?

An EDMS can be implemented at any point in time. While you might experience a gap in time in which documents cannot be retrieved or purged if they were created and stored solely in a dynamic EHR environment, as a go-forward strategy, EDMS implementation can be planned. The first steps are to complete the forms and legal health record inventories, including a listing of every electronic document or form. Each format should be defined as an episodic document image to be captured at time of discharge and interfaced electronically into the EDMS. These documents represent the full LHR, which reflects the discharge state of the clinical information. Any amendments to these documents would be entered as late addendums to the legal health record through the functionality of the EDMS system.

How do we educate information technology staff, vendors, HIM professionals, and students about the importance of the use of EDMS technology?

AHIMA offers a series of practice briefs and tool kits (see appendices) relative to electronic document management; these, combined with this book, can be used as tools to help encourage facilities to migrate toward the implementation of the EDMS as a complementary and critical component to the overall EHR. This journey is the same journey healthcare facilities took as they migrated from radiology file rooms to picture archival communications (PAC) systems as an adjunct component to radiology information systems (RISs). As the message becomes clearer in the industry concerning the importance of a working EDMS—via educational seminars, publications, and case studies—the evolution from paper to hybrid to electronic records will benefit from the strategy of Level 3 EDMS implementation.

How has point-of-service scanning impacted utilizing an EDMS?

Point-of-service scanning can be helpful in specific situations to speed up entry into the electronic record. For example, scanning consent forms, advanced directive papers, drivers license, or orders (if received in paper form) at point of registration can make these items immediately available across the enterprise. Scanning this information concurrently also saves time at post-discharge processing for the HIM staff who can then focus on clinical document scanning.

The author does not recommend point-of-service scanning in the actual patient care areas for clinical documentation because scanning is a secondary function to patient care activities and may not receive proper priority in processing. Point-of-service scanning on clinical units does not necessarily help increase efficiencies at the point of care. In fact, because of the production of interim or preliminary results reporting, multiple copies of documents can accidentally get scanned, creating more labor to remove the extra copies than would be needed to simply keep all scannable documents together and let the processing occur post discharge.

How helpful is backscanning of historical medical records when adopting an EDMS technology?

In most cases, based on the author's experience, the costs and labor to backscan records outweighs the benefits gained. Attempting to index documents that are scanned without proper forms identification—most likely absent prior to an EDMS implementation—can also add to the labor demand. Using a scan-forward methodology offers a more effective approach since it operates under the premise that as a patient is readmitted to a facility, the older records are scanned and made digitally available to the caregivers on a just-in-time basis.

The incidence of an adult patient returning to a facility after having been treated more than one time is more likely than the return of a patient that has not been back in a number of years. A common rule of thumb used by HIM professionals is that if an adult patient has had no activity at a health organization within three years, the likelihood of that patient returning for additional care is minimal. Newborn and pediatric patients may not return for many years due to the differing nature of healthcare in this population.

Are there any other long term risks to not implementing an EDMS?

Chapter 7 discusses one of the potential long-term problems: the inability to properly archive complete elements of documentation from an EHR if the LHR is not maintained within the EDMS. However, an even larger technical problem may occur if the LHR is not housed within the EDMS completely, particularly if the EHR software is replaced or upgraded. The upgrade or replacement process can make components of the records unavailable as part of a unified and complete legal health record during the release of information process as they may not be able to be transferred into a partial EDMS record that contains only scanned images.

Retention guidelines in a facility may be 30 years or longer, with some records requiring permanent retention. If all documents are not kept in a single document management environment and are instead retrieved via template reports and then combined with other electronically fed or scanned documents in other repositories, the records can no longer be easily managed, retrieved, and printed as may be required for legal purposes. Future technology compatibility and accessibility cannot be predicted, and therefore facilities open themselves to an incumbent risk if they cannot guarantee longevity of recordkeeping for legal purposes in an electronic environment.

For example, imagine a situation in which a part of a song was kept on a cassette tape, another part on a CD, and another on a vinyl record. Without the entire song being on a single technology platform, retrieving the song and piecing it together with the same output quality or in the same format, in a timely manner, would be difficult, or in the worst case scenario, impossible. It is better to maintain an environment designed to completely support LHR management of all EHR documents than to attempt to utilize a system that was designed for discrete data recording and reporting.

REFERENCE

HCPro. 2013 (October). EHR benchmark survey. *Medical Records Briefing* 28(10): 5, 7.

Abstracting: 1. The process of extracting information from a document to create a brief summary of a patient's illness, treatment, and outcome. 2. The process of extracting elements of data from a source document or database and entering them into an automated system.

Access: 1. The ability of a subject to view, change, or communicate with an object in a computer system. 2. As amended by HITECH, the ability or means necessary to read, write, modify, or communicate data/information or otherwise use any system resource (45 CFR 164.304 2003).

Access control: 1. A computer software program designed to prevent unauthorized use of an information resource. 2. As amended by HITECH, a technical safeguard that requires a covered entity must in accordance with 164.306(a)(1) implement technical policies and procedures for electronic information systems that maintain electronic protected health information to allow access only to those persons or software programs that have been granted access rights as specified in 164.308(a)(4) (45 CFR 164.312 2003).

Account number: A unique identification number associated with a patient and date of service used to delineate and access a specific episode of care. Also called Encounter number or Billing number.

Accountable care organization (ACO): A legal entity that is recognized and authorized under applicable state, federal, or tribal law, is identified by a Taxpayer Identification Number (TIN), and is formed by one or more ACO participant(s) that is (are) defined at 425.102(a) and may also include any other ACO participants described at 425.102(b) (42 CFR 425.20 2011).

Accreditation: 1. A voluntary process of institutional or organizational review in which a quasi-independent body created for this purpose periodically evaluates the quality of the entity's work against pre-established written criteria. 2. A determination by an accrediting body that an eligible organization, network, program, group, or individual complies with applicable standards. 3. The act of granting approval to a healthcare organization based on whether the organization has met a set of voluntary standards developed by an accreditation agency.

Accreditation standards: Pre-established statements of the criteria against which the performance of participating healthcare organizations will be assessed during a voluntary accreditation.

Active record: A health record of an individual who is a currently hospitalized inpatient or an outpatient. Also known as a clinical record.

Acute-care hospital: Under HITECH specific to the Medicaid program, a healthcare facility (1) where the average length of patient stay is 25 days or fewer; and (2) with a CMS certification number (previously known as the Medicare provider number) that has the last four digits in the series 0001–0879 or 1300–1399 (42 CFR 495.302 2012).

Addendum: A late entry added to a health record to provide additional information in conjunction with a previous entry. The late entry should be timely and bear the current date and reason for the additional information being added to the health record.

Admission date: 1. The date the patient was admitted for inpatient care, outpatient service, or start of care. 2. In the inpatient hospital setting, the admission date is the hospital's formal acceptance of a patient who is to receive healthcare services while receiving room, board, and continuous nursing services (CMS 2013).

Admission-discharge-transfer (ADT): The name given to software systems used in healthcare facilities that register and track patients from admission through discharge including transfers; usually interfaced with other systems used throughout a facility such as an electronic health record or lab information system.

Admitting diagnosis: The condition identified by the physician at the time of the patient's admission requiring hospitalization (CMS 2004).

ADT: Admission, Discharge, and Transfer software, which typically includes functionality such as Patient Access, Scheduling, Precertification, Bed Control, Master Patient Index, Transfer, and Discharge processes.

Advance beneficiary notice (ABN): A notice that a doctor or supplier should give a Medicare beneficiary when furnishing an item or service for which Medicare is expected to deny payment. If you do not get an ABN before you get the service from your doctor or supplier, and Medicare does not pay for it, then you probably do not have to pay for it (CMS 2013).

Advance directive: A legal, written document that describes the patient's preferences regarding future healthcare or stipulates the person who is authorized to make medical decisions in the event the patient is incapable of communicating his or her preferences.

Affordable Care Act: A federal statute that was signed into law on March 23, 2010. Along with the Health Care and Education Reconciliation Act of 2010 (signed into law on March 30, 2010), the act is the product of the healthcare reform agenda of the Democratic 111th Congress and the Obama administration (PPACA 2010); also called Patient Protection and Affordable Care Act (PPACA).

Alert: A software-generated warning that is based on a set of clinical rules built in to a healthcare information system.

All patient refined diagnosis-related groups (APR-DRGs): An expansion of the inpatient classification system that includes four distinct subclasses (minor, moderate, major, and extreme) based on the severity of the patient's illness.

Ambulatory care: Preventive or corrective healthcare services provided on a nonresident basis in a provider's office, clinic setting, or hospital outpatient setting.

American Health Information Management Association (AHIMA): The professional membership organization for managers of health record services and healthcare information systems as well as coding services; provides accreditation, advocacy, certification, and educational services.

American Society for Testing and Materials (ASTM) International: An international organization whose purpose is to establish standards on materials, products, systems, and services (ASTM 2013).

Analysis: Review of health record for proper documentation and adherence to regulatory and accreditation standards.

Ancillary services: 1. Tests and procedures ordered by a physician to provide information for use in patient diagnosis or treatment. 2. Professional healthcare services such as radiology, laboratory, or physical therapy.

Append: The operation that results in adding information to documentation already in existence.

Architecture: The configuration, structure, and relationships of hardware (the machinery of the computer including input/output devices, storage devices, and so on) in an information system.

Archival database: A historical copy of a database that is saved at a particular point in time. It is used to recover and restore the information in the database.

Archive file: A file in a collection of files reserved for later research or verification for the purposes of security, legal processes, or backup.

Assembly: Placing the individual paper or electronic documents within a medical record in a certain sequential order by category of form; most commonly reverse chronological or chronological order.

Attending physician: The physician primarily responsible for the care and treatment of a patient.

Attestation: The act of applying an electronic signature to the content showing authorship and legal responsibility for a particular unit of information.

Audit trail: 1. A chronological set of computerized records that provides evidence of information system activity (log-ins and log-outs, file accesses) used to determine security violations. 2. A record that shows who has accessed a computer system, when it was accessed, and what operations were performed.

Auditing: The performance of internal or external reviews (audits) to identify variations from established baselines (for example, review of outpatient coding as compared with CMS outpatient coding guidelines).

Authenticate: Confirm by signing.

Authentication: 1. The process of identifying the source of health record entries by attaching a handwritten signature, the author's initials, or an electronic signature. 2. Proof of authorship that ensures, as much as possible, that log-ins and messages from a user originate from an authorized source. 3. As amended by HITECH, means the corroboration that a person is the one claimed (45 CFR 164.304 2013).

Authenticity: The genuineness of a record, that it is what it purports to be; information is authentic if proven to be immune from tampering and corruption.

Author: Person(s) who is (are) responsible and accountable for the health information creation, content, accuracy, and completeness for each documented event or health record entry.

Authority: The right to make decisions and take actions necessary to carry out assigned tasks.

Authorization: 1. As amended by HITECH, except as otherwise specified, a covered entity may not use or disclose protected health information without an authorization that is valid under section 164.508. 2. When a covered entity obtains or receives a valid authorization for its use or disclosure of protected health information, such use or disclosure must be consistent with the authorization (45 CFR 164.508 2013).

Authorship: The origination or creation of recorded information attributed to a specific individual or entity acting at a particular time.

Backscanning: The process of scanning past medical records into the system so that there is an existing database of patient information, making the system valuable to the user from the first day of implementation.

Backward compatibility: The capability of a software or hardware product to work with earlier versions of itself.

Benchmarking: The systematic comparison of the products, services, and outcomes of one organization with those of a similar organization; or the systematic comparison of one organization's outcomes with regional or national standards.

Best of breed: A vendor strategy used when purchasing an EHR that refers to system applications that are considered the best in their class.

Best of fit: A vendor strategy used when purchasing an EHR in which all the systems required by the healthcare facility are available from one vendor.

Best practice: Term used to refer to services that have been deemed effective and efficient with certain groups of clients.

Bill hold period: The span of time during which a bill is suspended in the billing system awaiting late charges, diagnosis or procedure codes, insurance verification, or other required information.

Billing audit: See *Quantitative audit.*

Biometric identification system: An identification system that analyzes biological data about users, such as voiceprints, fingerprints, handprints, retinal scans, faceprints, and full-body scans.

Biometrics: The physical characteristics of users (such as fingerprints, voiceprints, retinal scans, iris traits) that systems store and use to authenticate identity before allowing the user access to a system.

Birth certificate: Paperwork that must be filed for every live birth regardless of where it occurred.

Breach of security: Under HITECH, with respect to unsecured PHR, identifiable health information of an individual in a PHR, acquisition of such information without the authorization of the individual. Unauthorized acquisition will be presumed to include unauthorized access to unsecured PHR identifiable health information unless the vendor of personal health records, PHR related entity, or third party service provider that experienced the breach has reliable evidence showing that there has not been, or could not reasonably have been, unauthorized acquisition of such information (16 CFR 318.2, as stated in Public Law 111-5 2009).

CDI: See *Clinical documentation improvement.*

Centers for Medicare and Medicaid Services (CMS): A federal agency within the United States Department of Health and Human Services (HHS) that administers the Medicare program and works in partnership with state governments to administer Medicaid, the State Children's Health Insurance Program (SCHIP), and health insurance portability standards.

Centralized HIM: The concept of work processes, equipment, and employees supporting multiple organizations from a single location. In a centralized HIM, staff is typically housed in an area that is located remotely from where care delivery is taking place.

Charge: In healthcare, a price assigned to a unit of medical or health service, such as a visit to a physician or a day in a hospital; may be unrelated to the actual cost of providing the service.

Charge capture: The process of collecting all services, procedures, and supplies provided during patient care.

Charge description master (CDM): See *Chargemaster*.

Chargemaster: A financial management form that contains information about the organization's charges for the healthcare services it provides to patients; also called charge description master (CDM).

Charges: The dollar amounts actually billed by healthcare facilities for specific services or supplies and owed by patients.

Chart: See *Legal health record*.

Chart management: See *Records management*.

Chart order policy: A policy that provides a detailed listing of all documents and defines their order and section location within the health record.

Chart reviews: Internal studies and external reviews including billing audits.

Chart tracking: A process that identifies the current location of a paper record or information.

Clinical abstract: A computerized file that summarizes patient demographics and other information, including reason for admission, diagnoses, procedures, physician information, and any additional information deemed pertinent by the facility.

Clinical analytics: The process of gathering and examining data in order to help gain greater insight about patients.

Clinical data analytics: The process by which health information is captured, reviewed, and used to measure quality.

Clinical documentation: Any manual or electronic notation (or recording) made by a physician or other healthcare clinician related to a patient's medical condition or treatment.

Clinical documentation improvement (CDI): The process an organization undertakes that will improve clinical specificity and documentation that will allow coders to assign more concise disease classification codes.

Clinical trial: 1. The final stages of a long and careful research process that tests new types of medical care to see if they are safe (CMS 2013). 2. Experimental study in which an intervention or treatment is given to one group in a clinical setting and the outcomes compared with a control group that did not have the intervention or treatment or that had a different intervention or treatment.

Coded data: Data that are translated into a standard nomenclature of classification so that they may be aggregated, analyzed, and compared.

Coding: The process of assigning numeric or alphanumeric representations to clinical documentation.

Coding and abstracting systems: Information system used to assign code numbers and enter key information from the health record.

COLD/ERM: See *Computer output to laser disk/enterprise report management*.

Compliance: 1. The process of establishing an organizational culture that promotes the prevention, detection, and resolution of instances of conduct that do not conform to federal, state, or private payer healthcare program requirements or the healthcare organization's ethical and business policies. 2. The act of adhering to official requirements. 3. Managing a coding or billing department according to the laws, regulations, and guidelines that govern it.

Components: Self-contained mini-applications that are an outgrowth of object-oriented computer programming and provide an easy way to expand, modernize, or customize large-scale applications because they are reusable and less prone to bugs.

Computer-assisted coding (CAC): The process of extracting and translating dictated and then transcribed free-text data (or dictated and then computer-generated discrete data) into diagnostic and procedural codes of varying classifications for billing and coding purposes.

Computer output to laser disk/enterprise report management (COLD/ERM): Technology that electronically stores documents and distributes them with fax, e-mail, web, and traditional hard copy print processes.

Computerized provider order entry (CPOE): Specialized software that allows clinicians to directly enter, authenticate, and date orders for testing, treatments, and other actions directly into software designed to process such orders; typically part of the EHR.

Copy/paste functionality: The act of copying text within the electronic health record, copying of text from an outside document and pasting it into the EHR, or pasting it to a new location with the record, in which the original text is not removed from the record.

Countersignature: Authentication by a second provider that signifies review and evaluation of the actions and documentation, including authentication, of a first provider.

Critical access hospitals (CAHs): 1. Hospitals that are excluded from the outpatient prospective payment system because they are paid under a reasonable cost-based system as required under section 1834(g) of the Social Security Act. 2. Under HITECH incentives, a facility that has been certified as a critical access hospital under section 1820(e) of the Act and for which Medicare payment is made under section 1814(l) of the Act for inpatient services and under section 1834(g) of the Act for outpatient services (42 CFR 495.4 2012).

Cross-training: The training to learn a job other than the employee's primary responsibility.

Current Procedural Terminology (CPT): Coding system distributed by the American Medical Association designed to be used as a tool for billing professional services in CMS Part B billing, as well as used for coding charge items and procedures in organizations performing CMS Part A billing.

Custodian of health records: The person designated as responsible for the operational functions of the development and maintenance of the health record and who may certify through affidavit or testimony the normal business practices used to create and maintain the record.

Dashboards: Reports of process measures to help leaders follow progress to assist with strategic planning; also called scorecards.

Data: The dates, numbers, images, symbols, letters, and words that represent basic facts and observations about people, processes, measurements, and conditions.

Data accuracy: The extent to which data are free of identifiable errors.

Data analyst: See *Health data analyst*.

Data element: 1. An individual fact or measurement that is the smallest unique subset of a database. 2. Under HIPAA, the smallest named unit of information in a transaction (45 CFR 162.103 2012).

Data integrity: 1. The extent to which healthcare data are complete, accurate, consistent, and timely. 2. A security principle that keeps information from being modified or otherwise corrupted either maliciously or accidentally; also called data quality.

Date of birth: The year, month, and day when an individual was born.

Date of encounter (outpatient and physician services): The year, month, and day of an encounter, visit, or other healthcare encounter.

Date of procedure (inpatient): The year, month, and day of each significant procedure.

Date of service (DOS): The date a test, procedure, or service was rendered.

Day outlier: An inpatient hospital stay that is exceptionally long when compared with other cases in the same diagnosis-related group.

Death certificate: Paperwork that must be completed when someone dies, as directed by state law; generally filled out by the funeral director or other person responsible for internment or cremation of remains and signed by the physician, who provides the cause of death.

Decentralized HIM: The concept of various work processes, equipment, and employees deployed to multiple locations, distinctly supporting multiple facilities.

Deficiency analysis: An audit process designed to ensure that all services billed have been documented in the health record.

Deficiency assignment: Each facility must develop its own procedures for quantitative analysis and responsibility for completion of the record must be assigned to each responsible provider; the deficiencies, or parts of the record needing completion or signature, are entered into the HIS or on paper worksheets attached to the incomplete, or deficient, health record.

Deficiency management: See *Deficiency assignment.*

Demographic information: Information used to identify an individual, such as name, address, gender, age, and other information linked to a specific person.

Designated record set: As amended by HITECH: (1) A group of records maintained by or for a covered entity that is: (i) the medical records and billing records about individuals maintained by or for a covered healthcare provider, (ii) the enrollment, payment, claims adjudication, and case or medical management record systems maintained by or for a health plan, or (iii) used, in whole or in part, by or for the covered entity to make decisions about individuals; (2) For purposes of this paragraph, the term means any item, collection, or grouping of information that includes protected health information and is maintained, collected, used, or disseminated by or for a covered entity (45 CFR 164.501 2013).

Diagnostic studies: All diagnostic services of any type, including history, physical examination, laboratory, x-ray or radiography, and others that are performed or ordered pertinent to the patient's reasons for the encounter.

Digital: 1. A data transmission type based on data that have been binary encoded. 2. A term that refers to the data or information represented in an encoded, computer-readable format.

Discharge: The point at which an individual's active involvement with an organization or program ends, and the organization or program no longer maintains active responsibility for the care of the individual. In ambulatory or office-based settings, where episodes of care occur even though the organization continues to maintain active responsibility for the care of the individuals, discharge is the point at which an encounter or episode of care (that is, an office or clinic visit for the purpose of diagnostic evaluation or testing, procedures, treatment, therapy, or management) ends.

Discharge analysis: An analysis of the health record at or following discharge.

Discharge date (inpatient): The year, month, and day that an inpatient was formally released from the hospital and room, board, and continuous nursing services were terminated.

Discharge days: See *Length of stay*.

Discharge summary: A summary of the resident's stay at a healthcare facility that is used along with the post discharge plan of care to provide continuity of care upon discharge from the facility.

Discharge transfer: The transfer of an inpatient to another healthcare institution at the time of discharge.

Discharged, no final bill (DNFB) report: A report that includes all patients who have been discharged from the facility but for whom, for one reason or another, the billing process is not complete.

Discrete data: Data that represent separate and distinct values or observations; that is, data that contain only finite numbers and have only specified values.

Document: Any analog or digital, formatted, and preserved "container" of data or information.

Document imaging: The practice of electronically scanning written or printed paper documents into an optical or electronic system for later retrieval of the document or parts of the document if parts have been indexed.

Document integrity: The process of ensuring all paper and electronic documents are received and included into a single medical record for each episode of care or visit and are equally accessible through a single request and purged with a single function.

Documentation: The recording of pertinent healthcare findings, interventions, and responses to treatment as a business record and form of communication among caregivers.

Documentation audits: Audits within the EHR that should look for completeness, timeliness, internal consistency, and other factors that have typically been evaluated in paper documentation.

Dynamic document: A template of discrete data elements that may be modified and displayed differently to an end user of an EHR, depending on the information and fields that are available at the time an electronic record is retrieved.

e-Discovery: The process of identifying content, format, timelines, or details about electronic documents within the legal health record that can be used for or against a defense in a case of negligence or fraud related to the patient care.

Edit: A condition that must be satisfied before a computer system can accept data.

Effectiveness: The degree to which stated outcomes are attained.

EHR: See *Electronic health record*.

Electronic Document Management System (EDMS): Software consisting of many component technologies that enable healthcare businesses to use documents to achieve significant improvements in work processes. Level 1 EDMS utilizes the scanning or document image functionality portion of an EDMS, but does not use complex workflow functionality or house the legal health record. Level 2 EDMS utilizes a greater degree of full EDMS functionality, including some workflow, but does not contain 100 percent of all source documents within the EDMS repository, leaving a fragmented electronic legal health record. Level 3 EDMS software, considered a best practice standard for HIM, supports organizations with complex workflow functionality, document imaging, indexing, archiving, and purging processes as well as complete integration with other source systems to maintain complete and functional legal health record within the EDMS system.

Electronic Health Information Management (eHIM). Typically used when describing transformation roles and workflow processes within an HIM department that is using either hybrid or fully electronic health records.

Electronic health record (EHR): An electronic record of health-related information on an individual that conforms to nationally recognized interoperability standards and that can be created, managed, and consulted by authorized clinicians and staff across more than one healthcare organization; also called computer-based health record, computer-based patient record.

Electronic health record management (EHRM): A generic term used within the healthcare industry to encompass the overall creation, processing, retention, release, archive, purge, and destruction of patient health record.

Electronic media: As amended by HITECH, (1) Electronic storage material on which data is or may be recorded electronically, including, for example, devices in computers (hard drives) and any removable/transportable digital memory medium, such as magnetic tape or disk, optical disk, or digital memory card; (2) Transmission media used to exchange information already in electronic storage media. Transmission media include, for example, the Internet, extranet or intranet, leased lines, dial-up lines, private networks, and the physical movement of removable/transportable electronic storage media. Certain transmissions, including of paper, via facsimile, and of voice, via telephone, are not considered to be transmissions via electronic media if the information being exchanged did not exist in electronic form immediately before the transmission (45 CFR 160.103 2013).

Electronic Protected Health Information (ePHI): As amended by HITECH, means information that comes within paragraphs (1)(i) or (1)(ii) of this definition of protected health information as specified in this section which is (1)(i) information transmitted by electronic media, and (1)(ii) information maintained in electronic media (45 CFR 160.103 2013).

Electronic record management (ERM): Systems that capture data from print files and other report formatted digital documents, such as e-mail, e-fax, instant messages, web pages, digital dictation, and speech recognition and stores them for subsequent viewing; also called computer output to laser disk (COLD) technology.

Electronic signature: A generic, technology-neutral term for the various ways that an electronic record can be signed, such as a digitized image of a signature, a name typed at the end of an e-mail message by the sender, a biometric identifier, a secret code or PIN, or a digital signature.

Electronic signature authentication (ESA): A system that requires the author of a document to sign onto a patient record using a user ID and password, reviews the document to be signed, and indicates approval.

EMPI: See *Enterprise master patient index.*

Encoder: Specialty software used to facilitate the assignment of diagnostic and procedural codes according to the rules of the coding system.

Encounter: The face-to-face contact between a patient and a provider who has primary responsibility for assessing and treating the condition of the patient at a given contact and exercises independent judgment in the care of the patient.

Enterprise master patient index (EMPI): An index that provides access to multiple repositories of information from overlapping patient populations that are maintained in separate systems and databases.

Enterprise-wide content management (ECM): Enterprise content management is a broad term used to describe the overall management of documents and data, typically in an electronic environment.

Episode of care: 1. A period of relatively continuous medical care performed by healthcare professionals in relation to a particular clinical problem or situation. 2. One or more healthcare services given by a provider during a specific period of relatively continuous care in relation to a particular health or medical problem or situation. 3. In home health, all home care services and non-routine medical supplies delivered to a patient during a 60-day period; the episode of care is the unit of payment under the home health prospective payment system (HHPPS).

ERM/COLD: See *Electronic record management.*

ESA: See *Electronic signature authentication.*

Feeder system: An information system that operates independently but provides data to other systems such as an EHR; also called source system.

File: See *Legal health record.*

Final note: A note becomes finalized either through attestation and system requirement or after a defined period of time, per organizational policies and procedures, applicable rules and regulations, and medical staff bylaws.

Flow chart: A graphic tool that uses standard symbols to visually display detailed information, including time and distance, of the sequential flow of work of an individual or a product as it progresses through a process.

Forms: See *Document.*

Format: Refers to the organization of information in the health record; there are many possible formats, and most facilities use a combination of formats.

Forms automation: The process of automating a paper form in a database so that the form can be printed from multiple locations throughout the organization and included within the health record.

Forms inventory: The process of gathering and strategically naming and numbering all documents that are designated to be part of the legal health record. The forms inventory includes a sample of all the forms from the output or printed perspective with each form, report, or document having a unique name or number.

Front-end processes: The billing processes associated with preregistration, prebooking, scheduling, and registration activities that collect patient demographic and insurance information, perform verification of patient insurance, and determine medical necessity.

Gap analysis: 1. A review of the collected literature and data to assess whether gaps exist. 2. Advice for those conducting the literature review on additional literature and data sources missed.

Go-Live: See *System go-live.*

Grouping: A type of software that assists in the process of dividing coded accounts into aggregate categories of classification to determine the prospective payment assigned to the specific case.

HDMS: See *High density mobile shelving.*

Healthcare: As amended by HITECH, means care, services, or supplies related to the health of an individual. Healthcare includes, but is not limited to, the following: (1) Preventive, diagnostic, therapeutic, rehabilitative, maintenance, or palliative care, and counseling, service, assessment, or procedure with respect to the physical or mental condition, or functional status, of an individual or that affects the structure or function of the body; and (2) Sale or dispensing of a drug, device, equipment, or other item in accordance with a prescription (45 CFR 160.103 2013).

Healthcare provider: As amended by HITECH, a provider of services (as defined in section 1861(u) of the Act, 42 U.S.C. 1395x(u)), a provider of medical or health services (as defined in section 1861(s) of the Act, 42 U.S.C. 1395x(s)), and any other person or organization who furnishes, bills, or is paid for healthcare in the normal course of business (45 CFR 160.103 2013).

Health information: As amended by HITECH, any information, including genetic information, whether oral or recorded in any form or medium, that: (1) Is created or received by a healthcare provider, health plan, public health authority, employer, life insurer, school or university, or healthcare clearinghouse; and (2) Relates to the past, present, or future physical or mental health or condition of an individual; the provision of healthcare to an individual; or the past, present, or future payment for the provision of healthcare to an individual (45 CFR 160.103 2013).

Health information exchange (HIE): The exchange of health information electronically between providers and others with the same level of interoperability, such as labs and pharmacies.

Health information management (HIM): An allied health profession that is responsible for ensuring the availability, accuracy, and protection of the clinical information that is needed to deliver healthcare services and to make appropriate healthcare-related decisions.

Health Insurance Portability and Accountability Act of 1996 (HIPAA): The federal legislation enacted to provide continuity of health coverage, control fraud and abuse in healthcare, reduce healthcare costs, and guarantee the security and privacy of health information; limits exclusion for pre-existing medical conditions, prohibits discrimination against employees and dependents based on health status, guarantees availability of health insurance to small employers, and guarantees renewability of insurance to all employees regardless of size; requires covered entities (most healthcare providers and organizations) to transmit healthcare claims in a specific format and to develop, implement, and comply with the standards of the Privacy Rule and the Security Rule; and mandates that covered entities apply for and utilize national identifiers in HIPAA transactions (Public Law 104-191 1996); also called the Kassebaum-Kennedy Law.

Health Level 7 (HL7): Founded in 1987, Health Level Seven International (HL7) is a not-for-profit, ANSI-accredited standards-developing organization dedicated to providing a comprehensive framework and related standards for the exchange, integration, sharing, and retrieval of electronic health information that supports clinical practice and the management, delivery, and evaluation of health services (HL7 2013).

Health record: 1. Information relating to the physical or mental health or condition of an individual, as made by or on behalf of a health professional in connection with the care ascribed that individual. 2. A medical record, health record, patient record or medical chart that is a systematic documentation of a patient's medical history and care and serves as the organization's evidentiary business record.

Health record analysis: A concurrent or ongoing review of health record content performed by caregivers or HIM professionals while the patient is still receiving inpatient services to ensure the quality of the services being provided and the completeness of the documentation being maintained; also called health record review.

High density mobile shelving (HDMS): Various configurations of movable and stationary filing systems that provide condensed storage of high volume materials such as paper medical records. Unique features of the system allow vertical storage through height of equipment, small footprint space for usage, and easy movement of shelving rows via electronic, power-assisted, or gliding carriages.

HIM: See *Health information management.*

History and physical (H&P): The pertinent information about the patient, including chief complaint, past and present illnesses, family history, social history, and review of body systems.

Hospitalization: The period during an individual's life when he or she is a patient in a single hospital without interruption except by possible intervening leaves of absence.

Hospital outpatient: A hospital patient who receives services in one or more of a hospital's facilities when he or she is not currently an inpatient or a home care patient.

Hybrid health record: 1. A combination of paper and electronic records; a health record that includes both paper and electronic elements. 2. Multiple electronic computer applications that exist which fragment the single legal health record.

ICD-9-CM: A classification system used in the United States to report morbidity and mortality information; International Classification of Diseases, Ninth Revision, Clinical Modification.

ICD-10-CM: International Classification of Diseases, Tenth Revision, Clinical Modification.

ICD-10-PCS: International Classification of Diseases, Tenth Revision, Procedure Coding System.

Implementation phase: The third phase of the systems development life cycle during which a comprehensive plan is developed and instituted to ensure that the new information system is effectively implemented within the organization.

Incomplete record processes: Processes including deficiency analysis and chart completion practices.

Indicator: An activity, event, occurrence, or outcome that is to be monitored and evaluated under the Joint Commission standard in order to determine whether those aspects conform to standards; commonly relates to the structure, process, or outcome of an important aspect of care; also called a criterion. 2. A measure used to determine an organization's performance over time.

Industry standard: The procedures or criteria that have been recognized as acceptable practices by peer professional, credentialing, or accrediting organizations.

Inpatient long-term care hospital (LTCH): A healthcare facility that has an average length of stay greater than 25 days, with patients classified into distinct diagnosis groups called MS-LTC-DRGs; prospective payment system for LTCHs was established by CMS and went into effect beginning in 2002.

Integrated delivery network (IDN): A group of healthcare providers and facilities working together within a single organization and group of leaders, typically in a single geographic region.

Integration: The complex task of ensuring that all elements and platforms in an information system communicate and act as a uniform entity; or the combination of two or more benefit plans to prevent duplication of benefit payment.

Integrity: 1. The state of being whole or unimpaired. 2. The ability of data to maintain its structure and attributes, including protection against modification or corruption during transmission, storage, or at rest. Maintenance of data integrity is a key aspect of data quality management and security.

Intelligent document recognition (IDR) technology: A form of technology that automatically recognizes analog items, such as tangible materials or documents, or recognizes characters or symbols from analog items, enabling the identified data to be quickly, accurately, and automatically entered into digital systems.

Interface: The zone between different computer systems across which users want to pass information (for example, a computer program written to exchange information between systems or the graphic display of an application program designed to make the program easier to use).

Interoperability: The capability of different information systems and software applications to communicate and exchange data.

JIT: See *Just-in-time training*.

Job description: A detailed list of a job's duties, reporting relationships, working conditions, and responsibilities; also called position description.

Job redesign: The process of realigning the needs of the organization with the skills and interests of the employee and then designing the job to meet those needs (for example, in order to introduce new tools or technology or provide better customer service).

Jukebox: A device used to store and retrieve multiple imaging platters or compact disks within certain systems.

Just-in-time training (JIT): Training provided any time, any place, and just when it is needed.

Key indicator: A quantifiable measure used over time to determine whether some structure, process, or outcome in the provision of care to a patient supports high-quality performance measured against best practice criteria.

Late reports: See *Loose reports*.

Legacy system: A type of computer system that uses older technology but may still perform optimally.

Legal health record (LHR): Documents and data elements that a healthcare provider may include in response to legally permissible requests for patient information.

Legal health record inventory: The process of identifying and logging the types, archived record discharge date range, and physical or electronic location of all records in a facility so that the records can be properly managed, including destroying them according to schedule.

Legibility: An aspect of the quality of provider entries in which an entry or notation is readable.

Length of stay (LOS): The total number of patient days for an inpatient episode, calculated by subtracting the date of admission from the date of discharge.

LHR: See *Legal health record.*

Longitudinal: A type of time frame for research studies during which data are collected from the same participants at multiple points in time.

Longitudinal health record: A permanent, coordinated patient record of significant information listed in chronological order and maintained across time, ideally from birth to death.

Loose reports: Documents, reports, images, or files that are received after the end of the patient visit or discharge and must be handled separately to be properly integrated into the medical record. Coding, billing, collections, and other processes cannot be completed until the full record is complete.

Machine learning: An area of computer science that studies algorithms and computer programs that improve employee performance on some task by exposure to training or learning experience.

Management: The process of planning, organizing, and leading organizational activities.

Mark sense: See *Optical mark recognition.*

Master patient index (MPI): A patient-identifying directory referencing all patients related to an organization and which also serves as a link to the patient record or information, facilitates patient identification, and assists in maintaining a longitudinal patient record from birth to death.

Meaningful EHR user (Related to Meaningful Use): Under HITECH, (1) Subject to paragraph (3) of this definition, an EP, eligible hospital, or CAH that, for an EHR reporting period for a payment year or payment adjustment year, demonstrates in accordance with 495.8 meaningful user of Certified EHR Technology by meeting the applicable objectives and associated measures under 495.6 and successfully reporting the clinical quality measures selected by CMS to CMS of the states, as applicable, in the form and manner specified by CMS or the states, as applicable; and (2)(i) Except as specified in paragraph (2)(ii) of this definition, a Medicaid EP or Medicaid eligible hospital, that means the requirements of paragraph (1) of this definition and any additional criteria for MU imposed by the state and approved by CMS under 495.316 and 495.332. (ii) An eligible hospital or CAH is deemed to be a meaningful EHR user for purposes of receiving an incentive payment under subpart D of this part, if the hospital participates in both the Medicare and Medicaid EHR incentive programs, and the hospital meets the requirements of paragraph (1) of this definition. (3) To be considered a meaningful EHR user, at least 50 percent of an EP's patient encounters during an EHR reporting period for a payment year (or, in the case of payment adjustment year, during an applicable EHR reporting period for such payment adjustment year) must occur at a practice/ location or practice/locations equipped with Certified EHR Technology (42 CFR 495.4 2012).

Measure: The quantifiable data about a function or process.

Measurement: The systematic process of data collection, repeated over time or at a single point in time (CMS 2013).

Medical necessity: 1. The likelihood that a proposed healthcare service will have a reasonable beneficial effect on the patient's physical condition and quality of life at a specific point in his or her illness or lifetime. 2. As amended by HITECH, a covered entity or business associate may not use or disclose protected health information, except as permitted or required (45 CFR 164.502 2013). 3. The concept that procedures are only eligible for reimbursement as a covered benefit when they are performed for a specific diagnosis or specified frequency (42 CFR 405.500 1995); also called need-to-know principle.

Medical record: See *Legal health record.*

Medical record number: A single unit number used to identify a patient uniquely within a healthcare organization within the master patient index. The eMRN (enterprise medical record number) is used as a single number within which to group multiple facilities' medical record numbers together. The eMRN is also unique to a single patient.

Medical specialties: A group of clinical specialties that concentrates on the provision of nonsurgical care by physicians who have received advanced training in internal medicine, pediatrics, cardiology, endocrinology, psychiatry, oncology, nephrology, neurology, pulmonology, gastroenterology, dermatology, radiology, and nuclear medicine, among many other concentrations.

Medical staff: The staff members of a healthcare organization who are governed by medical staff bylaws; may or may not be employed by the healthcare organization.

Medicare: A federally funded health program established in 1965 to assist with the medical care costs of Americans 65 years of age and older as well as other individuals entitled to Social Security benefits owing to their disabilities (CMS 2013).

Medication administration records (MARs): The records used to document the date and time each dose and type of medication is administered to a patient.

Medication list: An ongoing record of the medications a patient has received in the past and is taking currently; includes names of medications, dosages, amounts dispensed, dispensing instructions, prescription dates, discontinued dates, and the problem for which the medication was prescribed.

Metadata: Descriptive data that characterize other data to create a clearer understanding of their meaning and to achieve greater reliability and quality of information. Metadata consist of both indexing terms and attributes. Data about data: for example, creation date, date sent, date received, last access date, last modification date.

Method: 1. A way of performing an action or task. 2. A strategy used by a researcher to collect, analyze, and present data.

Microfilming: A photographic process that reduces an original paper document into a small image on film to save storage space.

Morbidity: The state of being diseased (including illness, injury, or deviation from normal health); the number of sick persons or cases of disease in relation to a specific population.

Mortality: 1. The incidence of death in a specific population. 2. The loss of subjects during the course of a clinical research study; also called attrition.

Natural language processing (NLP): A technology that converts human language (structured or unstructured) into data that can be translated then manipulated by computer systems; branch of artificial intelligence. Also referred to as computer-assisted coding (CAC).

Need-to-know principle: The release-of-information principle based on the minimum necessary standard.

NLP: See *Natural language processing*.

Numeric filing system: A system of health record identification and storage in which records are arranged consecutively in ascending numerical order according to the health record number.

Optical character recognition (OCR) technology: A method certain software uses to identify printed or cursive characters on paper documents or electronic scanned images created from the paper documents.

OMR: See *Optical mark recognition*.

Optical mark recognition (OMR): Also referred to as *mark sense*, OMR is the process of capturing data by requiring a page image to have high contrast and an easily-recognizable shape so that the page can be read by specialized software. A familiar example of OMR is the use of a number 2 pencil on a paper-based exam to provide markings that software can adequately identify.

Outcome: 1. The end result of healthcare treatment, which may be positive and appropriate or negative and diminishing. 2. The performance (or nonperformance) of one or more processes, services, or activities by healthcare providers.

Outlier: 1. Additions to a full episode payment in cases where costs of services delivered are estimated exceed a fixed loss threshold (CMS 2013). 2. An extreme statistical value that falls outside the normal range.

Outpatient: A patient who receives ambulatory care services in a hospital-based clinic or department.

Overlay: Situation in which a patient is issued a medical record number that has been previously issued to a different patient may be utilized by another patient; when portions of a patient's record get inserted in error into another patient's record.

Part-time employee: An employee who works less than the full-time standard of 40 hours per week, 80 hours per two-week period, or 8 hours per day.

Pathology report: A type of health record or documentation that describes the results of a microscopic and macroscopic evaluation of a specimen removed or expelled during a surgical procedure.

Patient: A living or deceased individual who is receiving or has received healthcare services.

Patient account number: A number assigned by a healthcare facility for billing purposes that is unique to a particular episode of care; a new account number is assigned each time the patient receives care or services at the facility.

Patient health record: See *Health record*.

Patient-identifiable data: Personal information that can be linked to a specific patient, such as age, gender, date of birth, and address.

Payment: As amended by HITECH, the activities undertaken by a health plan to obtain premiums or to determine or fulfill its responsibility for coverage and provision of benefits under the health plan; or a healthcare provider or health plan to obtain or provide reimbursement for the provision of healthcare (45 CFR 164.501 2013).

Performance improvement (PI): The continuous study and adaptation of a healthcare organization's functions and processes to increase the likelihood of achieving desired outcomes.

Performance measure: A gauge used to assess the performance of a process or function of any organization (CMS 2013). In electronic software, performance measures may also be referred to as key performance indicators or KPIs.

Performance indicator: See *Performance measure.*

Performance standards: The stated expectations for acceptable quality and productivity associated with a job function.

Personal health record (PHR): An electronic or paper health record maintained and updated by an individual for himself or herself; a tool that individuals can use to collect, track, and share past and current information about their health or the health of someone in their care.

PHI: See *Protected health information.*

PHR: See *Personal health record.*

Physician–hospital organization (PHO): An integrated delivery system formed by hospitals and physicians (usually through managed care contracts) that allows for cooperative activity but permits participants to retain some level of independence.

Physician query process: The process by which questions are posed to a provider to obtain additional, clarifying documentation to improve the specificity and completeness of the data used to assign diagnosis and procedure codes in the patient's health record.

Physician's orders: A physician's computer-generated, written, or verbal instructions to the other caregivers involved in a patient's care.

Point of care (POC): The place or location where the physician administers services to the patient.

Policies: 1. Governing principles that describe how a department or an organization is supposed to handle a specific situation or execute a specific process. 2. Binding contracts issued by a healthcare insurance company to an individual or group in which the company promises to pay for healthcare to treat illness or injury; such contracts may also be referred to as health plan agreements and evidence of coverage.

Post discharge: The time period that begins immediately following the conclusion of the episode of care. For inpatients, this time period begins at the time of discharge. For outpatient care, regardless of type, this time period begins with the end of the visit.

Prepping: The process used in document management to prepare paper records for scanning, indexing and quality-checking. Typically, prepping includes physically repairing pages, taping problem documents, staple removal, assembling the record based on designated sequencing and grouping like documents into a pre-prescribed order, and ensuring correct demographic data appears on each document prior to the imaging process.

Privacy: The quality or state of being hidden from, or undisturbed by, the observation or activities of other persons, or freedom from unauthorized intrusion; in healthcare-related contexts, the right of a patient to control disclosure of protected health information.

Problem list: A list of illnesses, injuries, and other factors that affect the health of an individual patient, usually identifying the time of occurrence or identification and resolution; see *patient summary*; *summary list*.

Procedure: 1. A document that describes the steps involved in performing a specific function. 2. An action of a medical professional for treatment or diagnosis of a medical condition. 3. The steps taken to implement a policy; see also *surgical procedure*.

Process: A systematic series of actions taken to create a product or service.

Protected health information (PHI): As amended by HITECH, individually identifiable health information: (1) Except as provided in paragraph (2) of this definition, that is: (i) transmitted by electronic media; (ii) maintained in electronic media; or (iii) transmitted or maintained in any other form or medium. (2) Protected health information excludes individually identifiable health information: (i) in education records covered by the Family Educational Rights and Privacy Act, as amended, 20 U.S.C. 1232g; (ii) in records described at 20 U.S.C. 1232g(a)(4)(B)(iv); (iii) in employment records held by a covered entity in its role as employer; and (iv) regarding a person who has been deceased for more than 50 years (45 CFR 160.103 2013).

Purged records: Patient health records that have been removed from the active file area.

Qualitative standards: Service standards in the context of setting expectations for how well or how soon work or a service will be performed.

Quality: The degree or grade of excellence of goods or services, including, in healthcare, meeting facility-set objective and subjective expectations for outcomes of care.

Quality check process: The process used in document management to provide a visual review of scanned and cold-fed documents for image problems, including illegibility, color intensity, image quality, redundancy or omissions.

Quantity standards: A measure of productivity performance based on x number of activities per y timeframe.

Queue: See *Workflow queue*.

Reassignment: Involves moving the document from one episode of care to a different episode of care within the same patient record.

Record completion: The process whereby healthcare professionals are able to access, complete, or authenticate a specific patient's medical information.

Record custodian: The person who has been designated responsible for the care, custody, and control of the health record for such persons or institutions that prepare and maintain records of healthcare. They are authorized to certify records and supervise all inspections, releases, or duplication of records. The custodian may be called to testify to the admissibility of the record, verify timeliness, and verify that normal business practices were used to develop and maintain the health record.

Record reconciliation: The process of assuring that all the records of discharged patients have been received by the HIM department for processing; in an electronic environment this includes the reconciliation of electronic files, reports, and records that may be COLD-fed from one system into another.

Records management: The overall process of creating, managing, modifying, completing, processing, reviewing, releasing, purging and destroying files.

Records purging policy: A policy that is used in conjunction with the off-site storage policy and retention policy.

Records retention policy: A policy that specifies the length of time that health records are kept as required by law and operational needs.

Re-disclosure: The release, transfer, provision of access to, or divulging in any other manner of patient health information that was generated by an external source to others outside of the organization and its workforce members.

Redundancy: As data is entered and processed by one server, data is simultaneously being entered and processed by a second server. The concept of building a backup computer system that is an exact version of the primary system and that can replace it in the event of a primary system failure.

Registry: A collection of care information related to a specific disease, condition, or procedure that makes health record information available for analysis and comparison.

Reimbursement: Compensation or repayment for healthcare services.

Release of information (ROI): The process of disclosing patient-identifiable information from the health record to another party.

Report: See *Document*.

Report cards: A mechanism to evaluate the quality of care delivered by health plans. They provide information on how well a health plan treats its members, keeps them healthy, and provides access to care (CMS 2013).

Repository: A data structure where data are stored for subsequent use by multiple, disparate systems.

Request for proposal (RFP): A type of business correspondence asking for very specific product and contract information that is often sent to a narrow list of vendors that have been preselected after a review of requests for information during the design phase of the systems development life cycle.

Scanning: The process by which a document is read into an optical imaging system; also known as document capture.

Separator sheets: Also known as lead sheets, these documents are used in the process of scanning as a type of cover sheet to identify a single or group of forms by category, within the document capture system when bar codes are not present on a document.

Service-oriented architecture (SOA): The policies, practices, and frameworks that provide the correct services or viewing of information and make information available at the time it is needed within whatever technology is being used. Service-oriented architecture is based on synchronization between the business and the IT implementation perspective. A well-formed service provides a unit of management related to business usage, and, when the service is abstracted from the implementation, one can consider alternative options for delivery and collaboration models between systems such as an EHR and an EDMS or an EHR and a PACS system.

SOA: See *Service-oriented architecture*.

Stable document: A document which, once created, cannot be modified in content except via annotation or amendment, and in which the original documentation element that was deleted, expanded, or changed, is also visually present to the reviewer of the document.

Stakeholder: An individual within the company who has an interest in, or is affected by, the results of a project.

Storage and retrieval: A healthcare facility's method for safely and securely maintaining and archiving individual patient health records for future reference.

Strategic plan: The document in which the leadership of a healthcare organization identifies the organization's overall mission, vision, and goals to help set the long-term direction of the organization as a business entity.

Subpoena: A command to appear at a certain time and place to give testimony on a certain matter; also called subpoena ad testificandum or subpoena duces tecum if record copies are provided simultaneously.

Superbill: The office form used for physician office billing that is initiated by the physician and states the diagnoses and other information for each patient encounter; also known as charge sheets.

System go-live: The date on which a software system is expected to be fully functional and made available to end users to utilize with actual patient data.

Team member: A performance improvement team role responsible for participating in team decision making and plan development; identifying opportunities for improvement; gathering, prioritizing, and analyzing data; and sharing knowledge, information, and data that pertain to the process under study.

Training: A set of activities and materials that provide the opportunity to acquire job-related skills, knowledge, and abilities.

Train-the-trainer: A method of training certain individuals who, in turn, will be responsible for training others on a task or skill.

Transcription: The process of deciphering and typing medical dictation.

Transfer of records: The movement of a record from one medium to another (for example, from paper to microfilm or to an optical imaging system) or to another records custodian.

Utilization review (UR): The process of determining whether the medical care provided to a specific patient is necessary according to pre-established objective screening criteria at time frames specified in the organization's utilization management plan.

Virtual HIM department: A theory of HIM management that proposes maintaining a minimal presence of HIM staff at the point of service location for patient care and providing a just-in-time approach to processing of electronic health records. The virtual HIM department typically uses the centralized HIM department infrastructure approach and increased numbers of remote workers.

Visit: A single encounter with a healthcare professional that includes all of the services supplied during the encounter.

Workflow: Any work process that must be handled by more than one person.

Workflow queue: A designated cache of electronically routed accounts that are assigned to a user based on predefined criteria that allow cases to automatically display sequentially to the end user.

Workflow routing list: See *Workflow queue.*

Zero charge case: An account that has been created in the master patient index (MPI), but does not contain any charges due to lack of an actual patient visit occurring, and therefore must be zeroed out and cancelled or removed from the MPI.

REFERENCES

42 CFR 405.500. 60 FR 63175. 1995 (Dec. 9).

42 CFR 425.20. 76 FR 67973. 2011 (Nov. 2).

42 CFR 495.302. 75 FR 44565. 2010 (July 28), as amended at 77 FR 54160, 2012 (Sept. 4).

42 CFR 495.4. 75 FR 44565. 2010 (July 28), as amended at 77 FR 54148, 2012 (Sept. 4).

45 CFR 160.103. 65 FR 82798. 2000 (Dec. 28), as amended at 78 FR 5687, 2013 (Jan. 25).

45 CFR 162.103. 65 FR 50357. 2000 (Aug. 17), as amended at 77 FR 54360 2012 (Sept. 5).

45 CFR 164.304. 68 FR 8376. 2003 (Feb. 20), as amended at 78 FR 5693, 2013 (Jan. 25).

45 CFR 164.312. 68 FR 8376. 2003 (Feb. 20), as amended at 78 FR 5694, 2013 (Jan. 25).

45 CFR 164.501. 65 FR 82802. 2000 (Dec. 28), as amended at 78 FR 5695, 2013 (Jan. 25).

45 CFR 164.502. 65 FR 82802. 2000 (Dec. 28), as amended at 78 FR 5696, 2013 (Jan. 25).

45 CFR 164.508. 67 FR 53268. 2002 (Aug. 14), as amended at 78 FR 5699, 2013 (Jan. 25).

American Society for Testing and Materials International (ASTM). 2013. www.astm.org

Centers for Medicare and Medicaid Services (CMS). 2013. www.cms.gov

Centers for Medicare and Medicaid Services (CMS). 2004. Regulations and Guidance. Transmittal 126, pg 6. http://www.cms.gov/Regulations-and-Guidance/Guidance/Transmittals/downloads/R126CP.pdf

Health Level 7. 2013. http://www.hl7.org/about/index.cfm?ref=nav

Patient Protection and Affordable Care Act. 2010. http://www.gpo.gov/fdsys/pkg/BILLS-111hr3590enr/pdf/BILLS-111hr3590enr.pdf

Public Law 104-191. 1996. 110 Stat. 1936. Short title see 42 USC § 201 note. www.uscode.house.gov/

Public Law 111-5. 2009. 123 Stat. 115. Short title, see 26 USC § 1 note. http://uscode.house.gov/

Appendix B: Managing the Transition from Paper to EHRs

The following originally appeared as part of the AHIMA Practice Brief entitled "Managing the Transition from Paper to EHRs" in November 2010. It was prepared by the AHIMA eHIM Workgroup and describes key best practice tips for managing transition into an electronic health record environment.

⊙ Managing the Change: Top 10 Paper/Hybrid/ EHR Tenets

1. The EHR must be part of an organization's vision and strategic plan. As part of this plan, the organization should have a standard definition for the legal health record.

2. The organization must ensure that adequate leadership, consultation, staff training, equipment, policies and procedures, and funding or other resources are in place to support EHR development.

3. Organizations must establish a legal health record steering committee to guide the organization from a paper to an electronic environment. This group must be empowered to make proactive and constructive changes. Its members should include department managers from health information management; risk, quality, or compliance management; medical staff; nursing; ancillary departments; IT, and the privacy officer.

4. The legal health record steering committee must develop and publish policies and procedures for operating in the paper state, hybrid state, and electronic state and include long-term archive, purge, retention, and destruction guidelines.

5. HIM professionals must participate actively in the development and implementation of the EHR, given the significant operational management effects on workflow within HIM and their role as custodians of the legal health record.

6. There must be a formal process for approving EHR software and hardware to ensure that it can support the organization's operational needs adequately for the paper, hybrid, and electronic medical record.

7. There must be a formal process for managing forms, paper, electronic, hybrid, and system-generated records, including input, output, and versioning of document content and access.

8. There must be a formal process and written guidelines addressing access, confidentiality, security, print control, spoliation mitigation, disclosure, and e-discovery.

9. A complete record inventory of all existing storage and management of paper, hybrid, shadow (duplicate), and electronic records must be maintained by all healthcare organizations.

10. The facility must develop a policy for retention and destruction of medical records, regardless of whether paper, hybrid, or electronic medical records are used.

The following table describes specific HIM functions, operational considerations, and suggested strategic guidelines for organizations to consider when planning the transition from a paper-based environment to a hybrid environment and then on to a fully electronic environment.

Strategic practice guidelines for traditional and emerging HIM operational functions

HIM Operational Function	Operational Considerations	Strategic Practice Guidelines
Transcription/ Coding Staffing	In-house, home-based, outsourced, or offshore	• Familiarize and synchronize transcription/ coding staff with your organization's strategic plan • Become knowledgeable about system integration capabilities, limitations, and opportunities of both source and interfacing information systems • Ensure availability and implementation of quality control features and reporting capabilities of all source and interfacing systems • Ensure compliance with any and all privacy, confidentiality, and security laws (e.g., state, federal, or organization specific) • Ensure organization has planned its off-site EHR content carefully before implementing any off-site coding or transcription functions (e.g., have major clinical documentation needed by coders, such as physician progress notes, available online to coders before implementing off-site coding) • Consider bidirectional interfacing for edits, changes, and other source document integrity • Consider electronic signature authentication; encourage online signature

HIM Operational Function	Operational Considerations	Strategic Practice Guidelines
Transcription Delivery Media	Fax, tape, disc or CD, paper, electronic (e.g., batch mode, uploading, integrity maintenance)	• Standardize delivery media to minimize paper and/or duplicate delivery modalities • Ensure device availability (e.g., remote access) and notification to recipients of delivered electronic documents • Ensure proper privacy and security controls are in place regardless of media
Electronic Signature	Transcription and other critical EHR documentation	• Review and consider e-signature processing capabilities, limitations, opportunities (see practice brief: "Electronic Signature, Attestation, and Authorship") • Consider versioning control and replacement of temporary versus permanent (after review and authentication) document storage • Understand clearly the minimal operational workflow requirements for processing e-signatures when working with information systems and vendor representatives
Release of Information (ROI)	Customer service when ROI function is off-site or remote; electronic transfers rather than paper printing	• Consider expansion of HIM responsibilities for ROI functions into decentralized areas, including off-site clinics, if not already responsible • Consider how to continue to meet standards and laws if ROI function is decentralized (e.g., disclosure laws with respect to ETOH, HIV, and mental health; have HIM continue to handle all requests for amendments coming through ROI) • Consider whether HIM will continue to maintain oversight or be a subject matter resource to those managing ROI; consider centralization of ROI and other printing and access functions for greater confidentiality, compliance, audit control, and cost efficiencies • Ensure EHR plans incorporate ROI workflow capabilities both on-site and remotely (e.g., disclosure tracking and auditing capabilities) • Consider electronic rules and alerts on ROI requirements to allow for expanded delegation of ROI operational capabilities and responsibilities

(Continued)

Strategic practice guidelines for traditional and emerging HIM operational functions *(Continued)*

HIM Operational Function	Operational Considerations	Strategic Practice Guidelines
Record Processing	Completion, abstracting, assembly, indexing	• Establish business rules for online EHR viewing that are based on an individual's role and completion status of online document (e.g., ROI only sees complete online records) • Ensure EHR system capabilities to monitor and track record completion (e.g., online alerts to individual clinicians, aggregated management screens and reports for HIM) • Manage record completion business processes, regardless of where organization is along the EHR transition continuum • Transfer and/or retrain staff members for other operational areas (e.g., assemblers become preppers and scanners where imaging has been deployed) as the need to print and assemble paper-based records diminishes • Develop standardized assembly order based on user needs for printed EHRs (e.g., different EHR views may necessitate different assembly orders [lawyers, patients, etc.]) • Work with EHR vendor toward use of expert rules for automated abstracting, where possible • Ensure productivity standards are in place for all record-processing functions • Determine which information will be back-loaded into the EHR system • Ensure that the workflow and work routing support COLD electronic document/results feed is used to reduce dependency on manual scanning of documents
Data Management	Data quality and integrity	• Ensure backlogs are eliminated before any EHR implementation • Ensure periodic spot-checks are made to ensure data integrity within the medical record • Ensure daily reconciliation of all interfaces for exported and imported feeds to ensure integrity of the medical record • Ensure processing standards (availability standards) are maintained as immediately as possible seven days a week 24 hours a day via adequate processing, staffing, and backups • Develop and review a data dictionary

HIM Operational Function	Operational Considerations	Strategic Practice Guidelines

File Room	Define the file room in terms of where files are stored and whether scanned images are used (are files paper, electronic, both?)
	
	Need to consider staffing support for retrieval of older records for length of retention; records are used most heavily the first three years after discharge
		• Conduct an assessment to determine where along the EHR transition continuum your organization's current and planned state of the file room is or will be:
		  ◦ Paper-based health record
		  ◦ Shadow health record
		  ◦ Hybrid health record
		  ◦ Complete EHR
		• Consider logistically what kinds of HIM policies, processes, procedures, and management practices are needed as the file room transforms from a physical environment to a virtual operation:
		  ◦ Elimination of shadow records
		  ◦ Shelving and hard-copy paper folders or files stored in a fixed location accessed and managed by staff
		  ◦ Electronic records contained on a server managed by information technology business rules for access, retrieval, retention, etc.
		• Consider which file room operations may need to shift to ensure acceptable productivity levels (e.g., timeliness, accessibility, completeness) in a hybrid file room environment (e.g., combination of hard-copy records, scanned records, and data repository records):
		  ◦ List of functions
		  ◦ Hours of operation
		  ◦ After-hours access and backup
		  ◦ Staffing needs
		  ◦ Record control
		  ◦ Filing and indexing
		  ◦ Retention, purging, and archiving
		  ◦ Other

Dynamic Data Handling	Alerts, flow data, e-mails, e-logs, and practice protocols	• Determine whether dynamic data will be considered part of the legal medical record • Ensure proper security measures are taken to protect your PHI if dynamic data are being maintained at a remote community health information network location • Determine whether online alerts and associated audit information should be included as part of the legal EHR

(Continued)

Strategic practice guidelines for traditional and emerging HIM operational functions *(Continued)*

HIM Operational Function	Operational Considerations	Strategic Practice Guidelines
Data Integration Issues	System merges, conversion issues, and multiple EHR systems in a given environment	• Ensure appropriate quality control mechanisms are in place to ensure data integrity (e.g., enterprise-wide master patient index encounters or episodes as part of the overall IT conversion process) for multifacility and/or multidepartmental EHR system integrations • Ensure HIM plays a strong role in all quality control planning and implementation activities (e.g., audit reporting and monitoring)
Retention/ Destruction Issues	State and federal mandates, legal counsel recommendations, and system limitations and needs; e-discovery policies	• Conduct a compliance review to ensure current policies are up to date with all state and federal laws on retention and destruction • Ensure that your retention and destruction policies include the components of the legal medical record that are stored in nonpaper-based media (e.g., remote and local servers, tapes, film, fiche) if the legal medical record is defined as being in a hybrid environment • Ensure that EHR systems have the ability to retain and destroy health information in accordance with your facility's legal medical record definition (e.g., fetal monitor data)
Definitions/ Glossary of Terms	Varying definitions of original, legal, complete, or hard-copy record; business rules	• Define what a complete medical record is in a paper-based versus EHR environment (e.g., transcribed outpatient clinic notes)

Position Description
Electronic Health Record (EHR)/Electronic Document Management System (EDMS) Coordinator

Position Overview
This position requires hands-on project management of the complete spectrum of HIM EHR and EDMS activities that will support the HIM department. This position serves as the central communication point with the IT and clinical/ancillary departments, to identify, investigate, communicate, and resolve system or procedural issues.

Reporting
This position reports to the director of HIM. Close interaction with various vendor and consulting teams, and HIM/Hospital teams.

Experience

- Minimum 5 years of HIM operational experience
- HIM certification desired
- Bachelor's degree preferred
- High level of HIM system knowledge and HIS technical aptitude required
- Previous experience with EDMS preferred

Required Skills

- Ability to positively interact with many types of system users
  - Including physicians and IT staff
  - Comfort communicating with all user groups
- Strong project management skills including ability to identify and resolve problems that require great detail and organizational skills
- Good verbal, written, and computer communication skills
- Ability to master project management methodology
- Ability to the big picture while managing details
- Ability to lead change management
- Deep HIM expertise
- Familiarity with forms usage and clinical charting processes including CPOE
- Strong comfort level with computers and ability to master deep computer concepts
- Must be able to flex work hours and will require some travel between sites

Core Competencies/Tasks

⊙ Learn the deep functionality of the document management system and apply knowledge to HIM processes in order to provide input and management of its design/setup and testing

⊙ Manage the implementation project with help from consulting staff and implementation team

⊙ Learn to administer the system to new users

⊙ Assist in design and execution of system configurations and help to provide workflow training to other staff on system functionality

⊙ Identify, track, and resolve problems by acting as a central communication conduit for the project

⊙ Assist in design and execution of testing scenarios for initial go-live and ongoing system updates

⊙ Provide input and suggestions for continual improvement of workflow processes

⊙ Provide input into the continued refinement of operational benchmarks and help to measure effectiveness of system

⊙ Act as a knowledgeable resource on electronic HIM and the EDMS system for the entire enterprise by keeping current on literature and technical knowledge and help to educate others

⊙ Serve on multidisciplinary committees addressing the EDMS implementation

⊙ Serve as backup to the EDMS operations manager

Note: This position is an important member of the document imaging team and offers unique opportunities for professional growth and enrichment in a state-of-the-art environment. As an integral part of the team that is implementing EDMS as part of the enterprise EHR, this position will serve as a knowledgeable resource that helps to define and protect the intricacies of the Legal Health Record (LHR) and continually reinforce education to others on the differences between HIM's electronic document management system and other patient-care-based clinical EHR sub-systems.

Position Description
Electronic Health Record (EHR)/Electronic Document Management System (EDMS) Centralized HIM Operations Manager

Position Overview
This position includes direct management and administration of EDMS-centralized scanning, prepping, quality assurance, release of information, and archival record functions, insuring efficient, productive, and high-quality system operations.

Reporting
This position reports to the director of HIM. Close interaction with various vendor and consulting teams, and HIM/hospital teams.

Experience

- Minimum 5 years of HIM progressive management experience and HIM certification
- Bachelor's degree preferred
- Good oral and written communication skills
- Basic computer skills

Required Skills

- Ability to positively interact with many types of employee and system users
  - Including physicians and IT staff
  - Comfort communicating with all groups who provide requests for use of medical records
- Strong project management skills including ability to identify and resolve problems that require interpersonal and organizational skills
- Good verbal, written, and computer communication skills
- Ability to see the big picture while managing details
- Ability to lead change management
- Deep HIM expertise
- Strong comfort level with computers and electronic workflow
- Ability to think outside the box to create innovative solutions to old work processes
- Ability to manage large groups of diverse employees across multiple work shifts
- Must be able to flex work hours and will require some travel between sites
- Ability to bend, walk, and lift up to 60 pounds on a regular basis, since working in an archival file area requires shifting of records and potential crank use in mechanical files
- Must demonstrate excellent knowledge of HIPAA and other privacy regulations and release of information standards, and expertise in archival filing system methodologies

Core Competencies

- Daily management of document management processes, including daily chart reconciliation, prep, index, scan, and quality control
- Management of interface capture and daily reconciliation
- Management of loose reports and other file and retrieval processes of paper and electronic records within scope of duties
- Daily personnel and budget management as required
- Management of the courier process
- Management of the request for information process
- Knows the deep functionality of the document management system and applies knowledge to HIM processes in order to provide input and management of its design, setup, and testing
- Identify, track, communicate, and resolve problems related to the operational areas
- Assist in design and execution of testing scenarios for initial go live and ongoing system updates
- Provide input and suggestions for continual improvement of workflow processes
- Provide input into the continued refinement of operational benchmarks and help to measure effectiveness of system
- Act as a knowledgeable resource on electronic HIM and the EDMS system for the entire enterprise by keeping current on literature and technical knowledge and help to educate others
- Serve as backup resource to the EDMS Project Coordinator

Position Description
HIM Data Integrity Coordinator

Position Overview

This position is responsible for insuring data integrity within the HIM department for (a) EDMS centralized scanning, prepping, quality assurance, release of information, and archival record functions, insuring efficient, productive, and high-quality system operations through measuring staff productivity and quality of output and (b) insuring that the data flow within the master patient index and legal health record is accurate and compliant with UHDDS and other data standards.

Reporting

This position reports to the director of HIM. Close interaction with various vendor and consulting teams and HIM/hospital teams.

Experience

- Minimum 3 years of HIM experience and HIM certification
- Bachelor's degree preferred
- Good oral and written communication skills
- Excellent computer skills

Required Skills

- Ability to positively interact with many types of employee and system users
  - Including physicians and IT staff
  - Comfort communicating with all groups who provide requests for use of medical records
- Strong project management skills including ability to identify and resolve problems that require interpersonal and organizational skills
- Good verbal, written, and computer communication skills
- Ability to see the big picture while managing details
- Ability to lead change management
- HIM expertise
- Strong comfort level with computers and electronic workflow
- Ability to work within Microsoft Excel and other databases
- Good understanding of statistics, metrics, and Lean Six Sigma
- Ability to think outside the box to create innovative solutions to old work processes
- Ability to manage large groups of diverse employees across multiple work shifts
- Must be able to flex work hours and will require some travel between sites

- Ability to bend, walk, and lift up to 60 pounds on a regular basis, since working in an archival file area requires shifting of records and potential crank use in mechanical files

- Must demonstrate excellent knowledge of HIPAA and other privacy regulations and release of information standards, and expertise in archival filing system methodologies

Core Competencies

- Development and implementation of daily chart reconciliation, prep, index, scan, and quality control mechanisms for all record processing jobs within the HIM department

- Management of interface capture and daily reconciliation and error resolution

- Manages error investigation and resolution regarding census and MPI data

- Daily personnel and budget management as required

- Knows the deep functionality of the document management system and applies knowledge to HIM processes in order to provide input and management of its design, setup and testing

- Provides input and suggestions for continual improvement of workflow processes

- Develops operational benchmarks and help to measure effectiveness of system

- Works with Coding manager to insure consistent reporting of quality indicators

- Works with any outsourced agencies on performance indicator reporting

- Acts as a knowledgeable resource on electronic HIM and the EDMS system for the entire enterprise by keeping current on literature and technical knowledge and helps to educate others

- Serves as backup resource to the EDMS project coordinator or operations Manager

Appendix D: Sample HIM Job Qualifications

Qualifications	Stages 0–1 Health Information Associate 1	Stages 2–3 Health Information Associate 2	Stages 4–5 Health Information Technologist 1	Stage 6 Health Information Technologist 2	Stage 7 Health Information Specialist
Education	High School or GED diploma required	High School or GED diploma, required; Some college preferred	Associate degree required; (BA degree a plus)	Associate degree in a related field required; or a Bachelor's degree	Bachelor's degree in a related field
Experience	Some general HIM experience preferred	1–2 years experience in a healthcare setting or related field preferred	2–3 years experience in a healthcare setting preferred	1–2 years in a healthcare setting required; 2–3 years preferred	2–3 years in a healthcare setting required; 4–5 years preferred
Medical Terminology	Basic skills preferred	Basic skills required	Basic skills required; intermediate skills preferred	Intermediate skills required; advance skills preferred	Advances skills required
Analytical Skills	Basic skills required	Basic skills required	Applied skills required	Advanced skills required	Advanced skills required
Problem Solving	General skills required	General skills required	Advanced skills required	Advanced skills required	Advanced skills required
Attention to Detail	General skills required	General skills required	Wide range of skills required	Wide range of skills required	Wide range of skills required
Computer Skills	Basic PC proficiency skills required	Basic PC proficiency skills required and basic skills in Word, Excel, and email preferred	PC proficiency skills required and basic skills in Word, Excel, and email required	PC proficiency skills required and intermediate skills in Word, Excel, and email required	PC proficiency skills required and advanced skills in Word, Excel, and email preferred
Content of Health Record		Working knowledge of the health record preferred	Detailed working knowledge of the health record required	Detailed working knowledge of the health record and chart organization required	Detailed working knowledge of the health record and chart organization required
Regulatory Standards		Working knowledge of privacy regulations preferred	Working knowledge of documentation regulatory standards preferred, detailed privacy regulations required	Detailed knowledge of documentation and privacy regulations required	Detailed knowledge of documentation and privacy regulations required

(Continued)

Qualifications	Stages 0–1 Health Information Associate 1	Stages 2–3 Health Information Associate 2	Stages 4–5 Health Information Technologist 1	Stage 6 Health Information Technologist 2	Stage 7 Health Information Specialist
English Language and Foreign Language	Written and spoken knowledge of the English language required	Written and spoken knowledge of the English language required	Written and spoken knowledge of the English language required and bilingual preferred	Written and spoken knowledge of the English language required and bilingual preferred	Written and spoken knowledge of the English language required and bilingual preferred
Keyboarding	General skills	Intermediate skills	Intermediate skills	Advanced skills	Advanced skills
Customer Service/ Communication Skills	Basic skills	Intermediate skills	Advanced skills	Advanced skills	Advanced skills
Specialized Skill Sets	Data analysis and research skills for error corrections preferred	Data analysis and research skills for error corrections required	Intermediate data analysis and research skills for error corrections required	Advanced data analysis and research skills for error corrections required	Advanced data analysis and research skills for error corrections required
Certifications/ Credentials			RHIT or other related credential preferred	RHIT or other related credential required, RHIA preferred	RHIA or other related credential required
Coding			Basic knowledge of ICD-9-CM (or ICD-10-CM/ PCS) preferred	Basic knowledge of ICD-9-CM (or ICD-10-CM/ PCS) preferred	Basic knowledge of ICD-9-CM (or ICD-10-CM/PCS) required
Hospital Systems/EHR Systems		Basic knowledge of hospital computer systems and EHRs preferred	Basic knowledge of hospital computer systems and EHRs required	Intermediate knowledge of hospital computer systems and EHRs required	Advanced knowledge of hospital computer systems and EHRs required

⊙ Sample Explanation of Level Expertise

Level 1, Health Information Associate I

Performs health information activities necessary to organize, maintain, and use electronic and paper patient health records. Depending on area assigned, may specialize in one or more clerical functions including: maintenance of records in centralized location; filing, indexing, and scanning; chart retrieval; and reconciling medical record activity. Accesses and updates electronic tracking systems. Answers telephones and assists with customer requests for medical records.

Level 2, Health Information Associate II

Performs health information activities necessary to organize, maintain, and use electronic and paper patient health records. Depending on area assigned, may specialize in one or more clerical functions, such as qualitative or quantitative physician documentation review and tumor registry support and follow-up. Responds to requests for information and serves as customer service liaison. Queries multiple electronic systems to locate requested information. Working knowledge of the chart organization, content, and external requirements related to chart documentation and privacy.

Level 3, Health Information Tech I

Performs specialized health information activities necessary to organize, maintain, and use electronic and paper patient health records. Depending on area assigned, may specialize in one or more clerical functions, such as coding clerical support, transcription processing and interface, coordination of record requests, image scanning quality auditing. Analyzes and researches errors. Participates in quality reviews. Compiles data and generates reports. Queries multiple electronic systems to locate requested information. Understands chart organization and content external requirements related to chart documentation and privacy.

Level 4, Health Information Tech II

Performs specialized or advanced health information activities necessary to organize, maintain, and use electronic and paper patient health records. Positions at this level have high customer service, strong analytic and problem solving skills, and require interpretation and explanation of policy and external requirements related to chart documentation, privacy, and release of information. Specific job responsibilities are based on the service unit assigned and include: release of information (ROI) to customers and patients, data integrity analysis and resolution (such as duplicate MRNs), analyzing and reassigning deficiencies when physicians are not assigned to the correct record deficiency, and assigning physician suspensions. Expert computer skills to navigate and query multiple electronic record systems.

Level 5, Health Information Specialist

Performs specialized or advanced health information activities necessary to organize, maintain, and use electronic patient health records. Positions at this level have high customer service and advanced analytic and problem solving skills; require interpretation and explanation of policy and external requirements related to chart documentation, privacy and release of information; and other departmental functions. Specific job responsibilities are based on the service unit assigned and include: release of information (ROI) to customers and patients, data integrity analysis and resolution (merging and unmerging duplicate records), and monitoring interfaces and working failure reports. Expert computer skills to navigate and query multiple electronic systems.

⊙ Sample Skill Gap Analysis Tool

This sample tool may be used in lieu or addition to any commercial survey tools utilized by the organization. This sample tool may determine the readiness of the employee to transition to the EHR environment.

POSITION TITLE:	Instructions for Rating Level of Experience		Instructions for Level of Competency
NAME: DATE: TEAM LEADERS:	Rate all Items in each core skill set below using one number (1–10) 1 = Minimal experience 10 = Maximum experience	Enter all your ratings (number or X) in the gray box	Put an X in the level of competency box that represents your level of competency for this skill set: Beginner = 1, 2, 3 Intermediate = 4, 5, 6 Complex = 7, 8, 9 Expert = 10

	Level of Experience	Level of Competency			
CORE SKILL SET	Min - Max 1 10	Beginning	Intermediate	Complex	Expert
Analysis/Testing	Example Rating: 4		X		
a) Performs detail analysis and data gathering b) Thoroughly analyzes and tests data to evaluate the effectiveness of systems and procedures c) Makes decisions and recommendations which reflect appropriate level of analysis and evaluation of options					

	Level of Experience		Level of Competency			
CORE SKILL SET	Min - 1	Max 10	Beginning	Intermediate	Complex	Expert
Specifications/Structured Design Methodology						
a) Formulates system scope and objectives through research, interviewing and fact finding for feasibility and completeness, identifying desired outcomes, requirements, and conditions of satisfaction						
Critical Thinking Skills						
a) Can identify major milestones and major or minor project deliverables						
Written Specifications						
a) Prepares detailed specifications from which vendor systems will be configured and/or programs written b) Prepares technical and user documentation						
Workflow Process/ Analysis						
a) Documents existing workflow processes and provides analysis to improve processes						
Documentation Skills						
a) Consistently and thoroughly documents and updates task statuses with detailed narrative on analysis, assignments, work completed, work to be done and communication with users. b) Prepares training materials.						

	Level of Experience	Level of Competency			
CORE SKILL SET	Min - Max 1 10	Beginning	Intermediate	Complex	Expert
Team Focus and Customer Service					
a) Participates effectively as a team member working collaboratively within the team. Demonstrates knowledge of and commitment to team goals b) Demonstrates flexibility and adapts to changing needs c) Presents a cooperative and helpful attitude at all times to internal and external customers					
Leadership and Communication					
a) Communicates appropriately with various constituencies to accomplish goals b) Effectively communicates with external and internal customers c) Accepts constructive criticism, adjusting performance/ behavior in response to such criticism					
Professionalism					
a) Represents Health Information in a professional manner, including demeanor, dress, code of conduct b) Acts as an ambassador for (employer name) while at work and at (employer name)'s sponsored events					

⊙ Sample Future State Questions for Staff Discussion

These are sample questions to solicit responses from staff during the initial planning phase for purchasing an EHR. After the initial implementation, HIM management may refer back to these questions as additional functionality is implemented within the EHR.

Script for HIM Director: *We will be meeting to discuss the future functions of HIM services. Please be prepared to discuss your thoughts. The following questions are a guide for this discussion.*

1. What functions do you think will be needed to support the electronic health record
   a. In the next year?
   b. 2 years?
   c. 5 years?
   d. Think about current processes; for example, will there be the same amount of paper to handle in 5 years?
   e. What new functions will need to be performed to support the electronic health record or other new functions?

2. In preparing your thoughts about the department, imagine that this is a brand new department to staff. Do not think of people that are already here, think of positions we need to perform the functions within an EHR.
   a. When will staff need to be at the hospital?
   b. What job functions will they need to perform?

3. Think about the new workflow for your area.
   a. What will be your workflow challenges?
   b. How would you like to solve them?

4. What is missing to achieve your goals?

5. Based on current statistics within your section, be prepared to think about the number of FTEs needed to do the new functions.

⊙ Sample HIM Department Future State Modeling Exercise

These are not recommended staffing standards; this is only an example of how you may assess the need in your department.

Current State Processes	Future State Processes	Positions Now	Positions Needed	Gap Analysis
Filing	No	6	0	−6
Chart Retrieval/Filing	Yes—temporarily	4	1	−3
Scanning QC/Prep Customer Service	Yes	2	8	6
Transcription Coordinator	Yes	1	1	1
System Maintenance—MPI/Physician Master/Guarantor Changes	Yes	1	2	1
Coding	Yes	15	15	0
Clinical Documentation Improvement	Yes	2	2	0
Analyst/Abstractors/Incomplete Records	Yes	6	5	−1
Transcription	Yes	22	24	2
Release of Information	Yes	3	3	0
Registries	Yes	3	3	0
Data Base Quality	Yes	1	1	0
Forms	Yes—some forms during transition and then focus on downtime forms	1	1	0
Security	Yes	1	2	1
HIM System Administrator/Analyst	Yes	1	1	0
Managers	Yes	4	5	1
Total		73	74	2

Appendix E: Fundamentals of the Legal Health Record and Designated Record Set

This practice brief originally appeared as "Fundamentals of the Legal Health Record and Designated Record Set." Journal of AHIMA 82(2) (February 2011): expanded online version. It was prepared by Mary Beth Haugen, MS, RHIA; Anne Tegen, MHA, RHIA, HRM; and Diana Warner, MS, RHIA, CHPS.

For years healthcare organizations have struggled to define their legal health records and align them with the designated record set required by the HIPAA privacy rule. Questions often arise about the differences between the two sets because both identify information that must be disclosed upon request.

The expanding scope of health records adds to the challenge of defining and compiling these record sets. An individual's record can consist of a facility's record, outpatient diagnostic test results or therapies, pharmacy records, physician records, other care providers' records, and the patient's own personal health record. Administrative and financial documents and data may be intermingled with clinical data.

In addition, the type of media on which information is recorded is also expanding. Source records may include diagnostic images, video, voice files, and e-mail. The organization must determine which of these data elements, electronic-structured documents, images, audio files, and video files to include.

The emergence of electronic health records (EHRs) also is complicating organizational efforts to define and disclose information. Information in EHRs is often stored in multiple systems, inhibiting the ability to succinctly pull together the record for either the legal health record or the designated record set.

These input systems may include laboratory information, pharmacy information, picture archiving and communications, cardiology information, results reporting, computerized provider order entry, nurse care planning, transcription, document imaging, and fetal trace monitoring systems, as well as a myriad of home-grown or individual clinical department systems.

However, the same criteria that organizations used to determine what paper records to retain and include in their legal health records and designated record sets can be applied to electronic records. Questions organizations must ask include:

- What information can be stored long term?
- What is clinically useful long term?
- What is the cost of storage?
- How can the organization effectively and succinctly assemble the EHR for long-term use?

This practice brief compiles and updates guidance from four previously published practice briefs to provide an overview of the purposes of the designated record set and the legal health record and helps organizations identify what information to include in each. It also provides guidelines for disclosing health records from the sets. The four original practice briefs are listed in the "Sources" section at the end of this practice brief.

⊙ Defining the Legal Health Record and Designated Record Set

There is no one-size-fits-all definition for the legal health record and designated record set. The healthcare organization must explicitly define both in a multidisciplinary team approach. Medical staff, for example, should provide guidance to ensure that patient care needs will be met for immediate, long-term, and research uses.✝[1]

In addition, organizations should consider the capabilities of their electronic systems, both immediate and long term. Additional considerations include ease of access to different components of patient care information and guidance from the organization's legal counsel considering community standards of care, federal regulations, state laws and regulations, standards of accrediting agencies, and the requirements of third-party payers.

Organizations should follow the following common principles when defining their legal health record and designated record set.

Legal Health Record Definition and Role

The legal health record serves to identify what information constitutes the official business record of an organization for evidentiary purposes. The legal health record is a subset of the entire patient database. The elements that constitute an organization's legal health record vary depending on how the organization defines it.

The legal health record is the documentation of healthcare services provided to an individual during any aspect of healthcare delivery in any type of healthcare organization. An organization's legal health record definition must explicitly identify the sources, medium, and location of the individually identifiable data that it includes (i.e., the data collected and directly used in documenting healthcare or health status).✝ The documentation that comprises the legal health record may physically exist in separate and multiple paper-based or electronic systems.

The legal health record serves to:

- ⊙ Support the decisions made in a patient's care
- ⊙ Support the revenue sought from third-party payers
- ⊙ Document the services provided as legal testimony regarding the patient's illness or injury, response to treatment, and caregiver decisions
- ⊙ Serve as the organization's business and legal record

---

[1] Throughout this brief, sentences marked with the ✝ symbol indicate AHIMA best practices in health information management. These practices are collected in the AHIMA Compendium (http://compendium.ahima.org), offering health information management professionals "just in time" guidance as they research and address practice challenges.

The legal health record is typically used when responding to formal requests for information for evidentiary purposes. It does not affect the discoverability of other information held by the organization.

When defining the legal health record, healthcare organizations should consider:†

⊙ The available functions in the EHR system that may generate relevant information. For example, does the EHR have clinical decision support, digital image import, or patient portals? Will information sent to or by the patient through the portal be inserted into the record and considered part of the legal record?

⊙ The storage capacity and cost for the required retention period of the health record. For example, what is the cost and storage capacity for WAVE files, transcribed records, and scanned documents or images?

⊙ The data's importance for long-term use. For example, organizations should define how to differentiate between different types of raw data. Some source documentation for test results, whether digital or paper, generally is considered useful only for short-term use (e.g., EEG tracings).

⊙ Whether the EHR system is able to provide both readable electronic and paper copies of all components of the legal health record.

Designated Record Set Definition and Role

The HIPAA privacy rule defines the designated record set as a group of records maintained by or for a covered entity that may include patient medical and billing records; the enrollment, payment, claims, adjudication, and cases or medical management record systems maintained by or for a health plan; or information used in whole or in part to make care-related decisions.

The designated record set also contains individually identifiable data stored on any medium and collected and directly used in documenting healthcare or health status. It includes clinical data such as WAVE files, images (e.g., x-rays), and billing information.

The designated record set is generally broader than the legal health record because it addresses all protected health information. While the legal health record is generally the information used by the patient care team to make decisions about the treatment of a patient, the designated record set contains protected health information along with business information unrelated to patient care.

Organizations must define the types of documentation that comprise the designated record set and identify where the records physically exist, such as in separate and multiple paper-based or electronic systems.†

Under HIPAA, the designated record set is used to clarify the rights of individuals to access, amend, restrict, and acquire an accounting of disclosures. Individuals have the right to inspect and obtain a copy, request amendments, and set restrictions and accountings of medical and billing information used to make decisions about their care.

⊙ Guidance for Defining Record Sets

The challenge for HIM professionals in defining the legal health record or designated record set is to determine which data elements, electronic-structured documents, images, audio files, and video files to include. The primary consideration in defining the legal health record and designated record set must always be the needs for immediate and long-term patient care. An HIM committee comprised primarily of patient care team members can guide this process. Members of this committee should make the decision on what information is clinically meaningful.†

1. Identify Relevant Regulations, Standards, and Laws

Based on the committee's clinical direction, the first step in defining the legal health record and designated record set is to determine what legal entities enforce relevant regulations, guidelines, standards, or laws on health records. Although these entities may have defined a legal record in paper terms (e.g., requiring a medication sheet rather than an electronic medication administration record), their definitions must become the basis for the organization's legal health record definition.

2. Determine Records Created in the Course of Business

The second step is to determine whether the records are created in the provider or entity's ordinary course of business. Source-system or raw data are the data from which interpretations, summaries, and notes are derived. They may be designated part of the legal health record, whether or not they are integrated into a single system or maintained as part of the source system.

Records from source systems may be considered part of the legal health record based on the content of the source system's record. Historically, reports or findings upon which clinical decision making is based are parts of the legal health record. For example, the written result of a test such as an x-ray, an ECG, or other similar procedures are always part of the record, whether these reports are integrated into a single system or part of a source system.

Working notes used by a provider to complete a final report are not considered part of the health record unless they are made available to others providing patient care. However, documents that are kept in a separate system (such as notes from a particular area of specialty that are kept separately but are treatment records) are always considered part of the health record.

The determining factor in whether information is to be considered part of the legal health record is not where it resides or the format it takes, but rather how it is used and whether it may be reasonably expected to be routinely released when a request for a complete medical record is received.

Uses of the information for business and legal purposes are usually, but not always, drawn from the legal health record. The most notable exceptions are those disclosures made for purposes of discovery or e-discovery in which any information requested under the court order must be provided.

Several states have laws or regulations that spell out the requirements and conditions under which health information from another healthcare organization or provider must be redisclosed. In the absence of more stringent state law, the HIPAA privacy rule prevails. However, because any medical or billing information that was used to make decisions about the individual is included as part of the designated record set under the HIPAA privacy rule, information must be disclosed or redisclosed if requested by the individual to whom it pertains, regardless of whether the information is external or internal.

3. Address Retention Requirements

The third step in determining the legal health record is ensuring that components are retained appropriately. Storing EHR components in disparate systems can cause problems. HIM professionals must identify and collaborate with IT professionals and system owners to define retention policies and practices. Without adequate retention of the EHR, compiling the complete record for release could be impossible.

A tool such as a matrix is critical for tracking the paper and electronic portions of the health record. As records are transitioned from paper to electronic, dates should be documented to provide a guide for staff when retrieving the patient's health information. (A sample matrix is provided in appendix A, Health Record Matrix.)

4. Consider How Data Would Be Produced

The fourth step in defining the legal health record and designated record set is to determine how information may be appropriately released. While it is easy to declare something such as an EKG WAVE file as part of the legal health record or designated record set, the organization must consider how it will be reproduced.

Questions to ask include if the source system can print or download to a CD, how it will be accessed by the requester, and if it will be in an understandable format. Components of the legal health record and designated record set must be reproducible in an accessible format. See appendix B for a comparison of the legal health record versus the designated record set.

5. Classify External Records

The fifth step is determining how to classify external records received by the organization. Some state laws address how to classify external records; however, in the absence of state law, the organization must determine if external records will be a part of the health record.

There is a school of thought that these external records cannot and should not become part of the legal health record because of the inability to attest to how they were originally created. To include them as part of the legal health record may result in implied liability for any inaccuracies the external records contain.

The opposing view is that if the external records were relied upon to make care decisions they should be included as part of the legal record. In addition, the College of American Pathologists requires that the laboratory director be involved with the decision on what lab results should be included in the EHR.

However, including external records as part of the designated record set and making them available in all appropriate disclosures, including disclosures in response to a subpoena, may accomplish the same purpose. The organization's legal counsel should be consulted prior to determining policy regarding the inclusion of external records as part of the legal health record.

Ultimately, the admissibility of the requested information in court is not the concern of the party producing the information. Compliance with the terms of the subpoena or order is required.

Additional Elements and Functions to Consider

As technology continues to evolve, other features will need to be evaluated and reflected in the legal health record and designated record set policies. Consideration needs to be given to documents that are not yet complete or in interim/pending status. Functions such as clinical decision support triggers and annotations need to be considered as well. Appendix C [...] lists the features and functions that should be evaluated when creating the policy for the organization's designated record set and legal health record.

Equally as important, organizations need to identify information that is not in the legal health record or designated record set. Data such as audit trails, metadata, and psychotherapy notes are not included in the definitions for these record sets. See appendix D for a sample list of items outside the legal health record and designated record set.

Other Federal Laws and Regulations

In addition to the HIPAA privacy rule, other federal laws and regulations give individuals the right to access their health information. Organizations must meet these obligations, as well as protect the confidentiality of patient records by ensuring they are released to or accessed by authorized individuals only.

The Privacy Act of 1974, like the HIPAA privacy rule, gives individuals the right to access and request amendments to their records. The act defines a record as "any item, collection, or grouping of information about an individual that is maintained by an agency, including, but not limited to, his education, financial transactions, medical history, and criminal or employment history and that contains his name, or the identifying number, symbol, or other identifying particular assigned to the individual, such as a finger or voice print or a photograph."[2]

The Medicare Conditions of Participation for state long-term care facilities state that the resident or his or her legal representative has the right to access "all records pertaining to himself or herself" including current clinical records.[3] In addition to clinical records, the term *records* includes all records pertaining to

---

[2] Privacy Act of 1974. 5 USC, Section 552A. Available online at http://www.justice.gov/opcl/privstat.htm.

[3] Centers for Medicare and Medicaid Services. "Part 483 Requirements for States and Long Term Care Facilities." Title 42 Public Health. Chapter IV. Available online at http://www.access.gpo.gov/nara/cfr/waisidx_01/42cfr483_01.html.

the resident, such as trust fund ledgers pertinent to the resident and contracts between the resident and the facility.[4]

The Confidentiality of Alcohol and Drug Abuse Patient Records regulation allows federally subsidized alcohol and drug abuse programs to give patients access to their own records, including the opportunity to inspect and copy any records that the program maintains about the patient. The regulation defines records as "any information, whether recorded or not, relating to a patient received or acquired by a federally assisted alcohol or drug program."[5]

The Occupational Safety and Health Administration requires employers to document certain employee injuries, including medical care provided in relation to those injuries. Employees and their designated representatives generally have access to such injury reports and related health records.[6]

The HIPAA privacy rule clearly indicates its intent is not to preempt other federal laws and regulations. Therefore, if an individual's rights of access are greater under another federal law, the individual should be afforded the greater access.

State Laws

Many states have laws or regulations that give individuals the right to their health information. Some state laws may define health information more broadly than the privacy rule. Some states may not limit access and amendment to PHI in a designated record set. When state laws or regulations afford individuals greater rights of access, the covered entity must adhere to state law.

⊙ Recommendations for Clarifying Disclosure

Healthcare organizations can take the following basic steps to help clear up confusion around the legal health record and the designated record set and the disclosure of information from both:

- ⊙ Develop and maintain an inventory of documents and data that comprise the legal health record. Consider whether other types of information that are not document-based are part of the legal health record (e.g., e-mail, electronic fetal monitoring strips, diagnostic images, digital photography, and video).

- ⊙ Develop a detailed inventory of items that comprise the designated record. Declare the official legal health record and designated record set in organizational policy.

---

[4] Centers for Medicare and Medicaid Services. "State Operations Manual: Appendix PP Guidance to Surveyors for Long Term Care Facilities." Revised December 2, 2009. Available online at http://cms.gov/manuals/Downloads/som107ap_pp_guidelines_ltcf.pdf.

[5] "Confidentiality of Alcohol and Drug Abuse Patient Records." 42 CFR Part 2. Available online at http://ecfr.gpoaccess.gov/cgi/t/text/text-idx?c=ecfr&rgn=div5&view=text&node=42:1.0.1.1.2&idno=42.1.

[6] Occupational Safety and Health Administration, Department of Labor. "Recording and Reporting Occupational Injuries and Illnesses." 29 CFR, Chapter 17, Part 1904.35, Section 657. 2002. Available online at http://www.osha.gov/pls/oshaweb/owastand.display_standard_group?p_toc_level=1&p_part_number=1904.

- ⊙ Consider a single repository for legal retention requirements.
- ⊙ Consider the use of records management software that supports the records declaration process and records lifecycle management, particularly for messaging records (such as e-mail or instant messages that are considered part of the legal health record or designated record set).
- ⊙ Collaborate with clinicians to develop procedures for identifying external information that has been used in patient care. Once identified as such, provisions should be made for including this in the patient's record, whether paper or electronic. Within the record, consideration should be given to filing or indexing the external information under a separate tab or section of the electronic or paper record developed for this purpose. Review state statutes that may require inclusion of external information.
- ⊙ Promptly return to the patient (if feasible) or dispose of (in accordance with the organization's destruction procedures) any health information that is not used or not solicited.
- ⊙ Consider developing policies and procedures that confine the ability to request health information from external sources and to place such information in the patient's record to specified staff or personnel.
- ⊙ Develop written policies and procedures as well as staff training for clinical users that address the use of external information. Train HIM staff on procedures related to redisclosure of health information.
- ⊙ Identify the records the organization believes individuals have the right to access and amend under state and federal laws and regulations.
- ⊙ Apply HIPAA's preemption standards where individuals' rights to access and amend are not the same under other federal or state laws and regulations.

There may be times when an individual has a legitimate need to access source data that are not considered part of the legal health record or designated record set. The organization's legal counsel should advise whenever there is uncertainty. Appendix E contains policy definitions that can be included in organizational policy. Appendix F offers a sample template for the legal health record, and appendix G features a sample template for a designated record set policy.

SOURCES

AHIMA e-HIM Work Group on the Legal Health Record. 2005 (September). Update: Guidelines for defining the legal health record for disclosure purposes. *Journal of AHIMA* 76(8): 64A–G. Available online in the AHIMA Body of Knowledge at http://www.ahima.org.

AHIMA EHR Practice Council. 2007 (October). Developing a legal health record policy. *Journal of AHIMA* 78(9): 93–97. Available online in the AHIMA Body of Knowledge at http://www.ahima.org.

Hughes, G. 2003 (January). Defining the designated record set. *Journal of AHIMA* 74(1): 64A–D. Available online in the AHIMA Body of Knowledge at http://www.ahima.org.

Dougherty, M., and L. Washington. 2008 (April). Defining and disclosing the designated record set and the legal health record. *Journal of AHIMA* 79(4): 65–68. Available online in the AHIMA Body of Knowledge at http://www.ahima.org.

⊙ Appendices

Seven appendices are included in this brief.

Appendix A: Health Record Matrix

The following matrix is a tool organizations can use to help identify and track the paper and electronic portions of the health record during an EHR implementation and ongoing maintenance. HIM professionals can customize this matrix to their organization's needs and add specific items that should be considered when implementing an EHR. It is up to each individual organization to determine what health information is considered part of their legal health record and their designated record set.

Type of Document	Name of Document	Primary Source*	Primary Source System Start Date	Source of the Legal Health Record/ Designated Record Set	Legal Health Record, Designated Record Set, or Both	Comments
Nursing	ICU nursing assessment	Electronic nursing documentation system	1/2/2007	Enterprise document management system	Both	Phased implementation
Physician orders	Congestive heart failure order set	Computerized physician order entry system	1/2/2007	EHR	Both	Downtime paper orders scanned
Emergency department	Emergency department treatment record	Paper	3/15/2005	Enterprise document system	Both	
Discharge summary	Discharge summary	Transcription system	12/15/2002	EHR	Both	
Claims	Billing report	Patient financial system	7/1/1998	Patient financial system	Designated record set	

*Includes scanned images

Appendix B: Comparison of the Designated Record Set versus the Legal Health Record

This side-by-side comparison of the designated record set and the legal health record demonstrates the differences between the two sets of information, as well as their purposes.

	Designated Record Set	Legal Health Record
Definition	A group of records maintained by or for a covered entity that is the medical and billing records about individuals; enrollment, payment, claims adjudication, and case or medical management record systems maintained by or for a health plan; information used in whole or in part by or for the HIPAA covered entity to make decisions about individuals.	The business record generated at or for a healthcare organization. It is the record that would be released upon receipt of a request. The legal health record is the officially declared record of healthcare services provided to an individual delivered by a provider.
Purpose	Used to clarify the access and amendment standards in the HIPAA privacy rule, which provide that individuals generally have the right to inspect and obtain a copy of protected health information in the designated record set.	The official business record of healthcare services delivered by the entity for regulatory and disclosure purposes.
Content	Defined in organizational policy and required by the HIPAA privacy rule. The content of the designated record set includes medical and billing records of covered providers; enrollment, payment, claims, and case information of a health plan; and information used in whole or in part by or for the covered entity to make decisions about individuals.	Defined in organizational policy and can include individually identifiable data in any medium collected and directly used in documenting healthcare services or health status. It excludes administrative, derived, and aggregate data.
Uses	Supports individual HIPAA right of access and amendment.	Provides a record of health status as well as documentation of care for reimbursement, quality management, research, and public health purposes; facilitates business decision making and education of healthcare practitioners as well as the legal needs of the healthcare organization.

Categorizing record types can assist in understanding the similarities and differences and help organizations develop policies for each. Some record types are found in both the designated record set and the legal health record, while others are specific to the designated record set. The following table provides examples of different types of records and shows the similarities and differences between the two sets of information.

Sorting Record Types

Some record types belong in both the designated record set and the legal health record. Some belong in the designated record set only. Categorizing record types helps organizations set policies for each record set.

Clinical Record	Source Clinical Data	External Records and Reports
• History and physical • Orders • Progress notes • Lab reports (including contract lab) • Progress notes • Vital signs • Assessments • Consults • Clinical reports • Authorizations and consents designated record set and legal health record	• X-rays • Images • Fetal strips • Videos • Pathology slides designated record set and legal health record	• External records referenced for patient care: other providers' records, records provided upon transfer • Patient generated records • Personal health records designated record set and possibly legal health record*

* There are two points of view on whether external records referenced for patient care are part of the legal health record. One view is that they should be if they were relied upon to make care decisions. The other view is that although they are part of the designated record set and are available for patient care and disclosures, they should not be because of the organization's inability to attest to how the external records were originally created. Organizations should consult with their counsels to weigh the risks and benefits of either approach.

Committee Reports (of Patient-Specific Care Decisions)	Administrative and Financial	Secondary/Administrative and Statistical
• Ethics committee or tumor board, if deciding on a course of treatment for an individual patient Note: Documentation of findings could be reported in the patient's medical record. Other legal privileges may apply to these records. designated record set only	• Super bills/encounter forms • Remittance advice • Case management records designated record set only	• Tumor registries data • QI/QM reports and abstracts • Statistical data • Committee minutes (not patient-specific treatment related) neither

Appendix C: Considerations for the Legal Health Record and Designated Record Set

The move toward electronic health records is complicating organizational efforts to define and disclose information. Many of the items within the EHR have not historically been included in the legal health record and the designated record set. Examples of documents and data that should be evaluated for inclusion or exclusion include, but are not limited to:

- ⊙ Administrative data/documents: patient-identifiable data used for administrative, regulatory, healthcare operations, and payment (financial) purposes.[7]

- ⊙ Annotations/"sticky notes": additional information that is added as a layer on top of the note. The annotation or sticky note may be suppressed when viewing or printing. These may be considered part of the health record. This documentation may become a permanent part of the record and is maintained in a manner similar to any other information contained within the health record.

- ⊙ Clinical decision support systems: a subcategory of clinical information systems that is designed to help healthcare professionals make knowledge-based clinical decisions.[8] Currently there are no generally accepted rules on including decision support such as system-generated notifications, prompts, and alerts as part of the health record.[9] Alerts, reminders, pop-ups, and similar tools are used as aides in the clinical decision-making process. The tools themselves are usually not considered part of the legal health record; however, associated documentation is considered a component.[10] At a minimum, the EHR should include documentation of the clinician's actions in response to decision support. This documentation is evidence of the clinician's decision to follow or disregard decision support. The organization should define the extent of exception documentation required (e.g., what no documentation means).[11] When an organization decides to include the decision support trigger as part of the health record, the organization will need to define if all triggers will be part of the record or just the clinical decision support triggers. For example, alerts for patient appointment reminders may not be considered part of the legal health record, but alerts for drug-drug interaction may be.[12]

[7] AHIMA EHR Practice Council. 2007 (October). Developing a legal health record policy: Appendix A. Journal of AHIMA 78(9): web extra. Available online in the AHIMA Body of Knowledge at http://www.ahima.org.

[8] American Health Information Management Association. 2009. Pocket Glossary of Health Information Management and Technology. Chicago, IL: AHIMA.

[9] AHIMA EHR Practice Council. 2007 (October). Developing a legal health record policy. Journal of AHIMA 78(9): 93–97. Available online in the AHIMA Body of Knowledge at http://www.ahima.org.

[10] AHIMA e-HIM Work Group on the Legal Health Record. 2005 (September). Update: Guidelines for defining the legal health record for disclosure purposes. *Journal of AHIMA* 76(8): 64A-G. Available online in the AHIMA Body of Knowledge at http://www.ahima.org.

[11] AHIMA EHR Practice Council. 2007 (October). Developing a legal health record policy. *Journal of AHIMA* 78(9): 93-97. Available online in the AHIMA Body of Knowledge at http://www.ahima.org.

[12] Warner, D. 2010 (March). Evaluating alerts and triggers: Determining whether alerts and triggers are part of the legal health record. *Journal of AHIMA* 81(3): 40-41. Available online in the AHIMA Body of Knowledge at http://www.ahima.org.

⊙ Coding queries: a routine communication and education tool used to advocate complete and compliant documentation. Retention of the query varies by healthcare organization. First, an organization must determine if the query will be part of the health record. If the query is not part of the health record, then the organization must decide if the query is kept as part of the business record or only the outcome of the query is maintained in a database.[13]

⊙ Continuing care records: records received from another healthcare provider. Historically, these records were generally not considered part of the legal health record unless they were used in the provision of patient care. In the EHR it may be difficult to determine if information was viewed or used in delivering healthcare. It may be necessary to define such information as part of the legal health record. Policies should reflect the proper disposition of health records from external sources (e.g., other healthcare providers) if they are not integrated into the electronic and legal health record.[14]

⊙ Data/documents: documentation of patient care that took place in the ordinary course of business by all healthcare providers.[15]

⊙ Data from source systems: written results of tests. Data from which interpretations, summaries, notes, flowcharts, etc., are derived.[16]

⊙ Discrete structured data: laboratory orders/refills, orders/medication orders/MARs, online charting and documentation, and any detailed charges.[17]

⊙ Document completion (lockdown): organizations must determine when users can no longer create or make changes to electronic documentation. Organizations with several source systems should consider locking down documents at some determined time after a patient encounter. There may be limitations with how the EHR handles this function, which organizations will need to factor into their policies.[18]

⊙ External records and reports: healthcare records that are created by providers outside of the organization that are received by the organization for patient care. The decision of which category external records and reports fall into depends on the applicability of HIPAA privacy rules, state law or regulation, source of the request, and type of request. If external records and reports are used to make decisions about an individual,

---

[13] American Health Information Management Association. 2010 (May). Guidance for clinical documentation improvement programs. *Journal of AHIMA* 81(5): expanded web version. Available online in the AHIMA Body of Knowledge at http://www.ahima.org.

[14] AHIMA e-HIM Work Group on the Legal Health Record. 2005 (September). Update: Guidelines for defining the legal health record for disclosure purposes. *Journal of AHIMA* 76(8): 64A-G. Available online in the AHIMA Body of Knowledge at http://www.ahima.org.

[15] AHIMA EHR Practice Council. 2007 (October). Developing a legal health record policy: Appendix A. *Journal of AHIMA* 78(9): web extra. Available online in the AHIMA Body of Knowledge at http://www.ahima.org.

[16] Ibid.

[17] Ibid.

[18] AHIMA EHR Practice Council. 2007 (October). Developing a legal health record policy. *Journal of AHIMA* 78(9): 93-97. Available online in the AHIMA Body of Knowledge at http://www.ahima.org.

they become part of the designated record set. If those decisions are care decisions, in most cases those same records and reports will also be included in the provider's legal health record, especially if they are created pursuant to a contract.[19]

⊙ Personal health records (PHRs): copies of PHRs that are created, owned, and managed by the patient and are provided to a healthcare organization(s) may be considered part of the health record if so defined by the organization.[20]

⊙ Research records: organizational policy should differentiate whether research records are part of the health record and how these records will be kept.[21]

⊙ Version control: organizations must decide whether all versions of a document or ancillary report will be displayed or just the final version.[22]

⊙ Diagnostic image data: CT, MRI, ultrasound, nuclear medicine, etc.[23]

⊙ Signal tracing data: EKG, EEG, fetal monitoring signal tracings, etc.[24]

⊙ Audio data: heart sounds, voice dictations, annotations, etc.[25]

⊙ Video data: ultrasound, cardiac catheterization examinations, etc.[26]

⊙ Text data: radiology reports, transcribed reports, UBS, itemized bills, etc.[27]

⊙ Original analog document—document image data: signed patient consent forms, handwritten notes, drawings, etc.[28]

Appendix D: Documents that Fall Outside the Designated Record Set and Legal Health Record

Editor's note: portions of this document were previously published in two practice briefs. The original practice briefs are listed in the "Sources" section at the end of this appendix.

---

[19] Dougherty, M., and L. Washington. 2008 (April). Defining and disclosing the designated record set and the legal health record. Journal of AHIMA 79(4): 65-68. Available online in the AHIMA Body of Knowledge at http://www.ahima.org.

[20] AHIMA EHR Practice Council. 2007 (October). Developing a legal health record policy: Appendix A. *Journal of AHIMA* 78(9): web extra. Available online in the AHIMA Body of Knowledge at http://www.ahima.org.

[21] Ibid.

[22] AHIMA EHR Practice Council. 2007 (October). Developing a legal health record policy. *Journal of AHIMA* 78(9): 93-97. Available online in the AHIMA Body of Knowledge at http://www.ahima.org.

[23] AHIMA EHR Practice Council. 2007 (October). Developing a legal health record policy: Appendix A. *Journal of AHIMA* 78(9): web extra. Available online in the AHIMA Body of Knowledge at http://www.ahima.org.

[24] Ibid.

[25] Ibid.

[26] Ibid.

[27] Ibid.

[28] Ibid.

In its definition of the designated record set the privacy rule does not specifically address source data such as pathology slides, diagnostic films, and tracings. However, narrative throughout the preamble suggests that providing interpretations from source data would generally be acceptable in the designated record set. In most cases, individuals cannot interpret source data, so such data is meaningless. On the other hand, the interpretations of source data provide individuals with information needed to make informed decisions about their healthcare.

There may be times, however, when an individual has a legitimate need to access source data. When such a need arises, the covered entity will want to provide the individual with greater rights of access, allowing the individual access to or copies of the source data when possible.

The following table provides examples of those documents that are not included in the designated record set.

Outside the Designated Record Set	Examples
Health information generated, collected, or maintained for purposes that do not include decision making about the individual	• Data collected and maintained for research • Data collected and maintained for peer review purposes • Data collected and maintained for performance improvement purposes • Appointment and surgery schedules • Birth and death registers • Surgery registers • Diagnostic or operative indexes • Duplicate copies of information that can also be located in the individual's medical or billing record
Psychotherapy notes	The notes of a mental health professional about counseling sessions that are maintained separate and apart from the regular health record
Information compiled in reasonable anticipation of or for use in a civil, criminal, or administrative action or proceeding	Notes taken by a covered entity during a meeting with the covered entity's attorney about a pending lawsuit
CLIA	• Requisitions for laboratory tests • Duplicate lab results when the originals are filed in the individual's paper chart
Employer records	• Pre-employment physicals maintained in human resource files • The results of HIV tests maintained by the infectious disease control nurse on employees who have suffered needle stick injuries on the job

(Continued)

Outside the Designated Record Set	Examples
Business associate records that meet the definition of designated record set but that merely duplicate information maintained by the covered entity	Transcribed operative reports that have been transmitted to the covered entity
Education records	Records generated and maintained by teachers and teachers' aides employed by a school district or patients in acute care hospitals, institutions for the developmentally disabled and rehabilitation care centers
Source (raw) data interpreted or summarized in the individual's medical or health record	• Pathology slides • Diagnostic films • Electrocardiogram tracings from which interpretations are derived
Versions	Management of multiple revisions of the same document; by versioning, each iteration of a document is tracked
Metadata	Data that provides a detailed description about other data; "Information about a particular data set or document that describes how, when, and by whom it was collected, created, accessed, or modified and how it is formatted"[29]
Audits	Results of reviews to identify variations from established baselines or used to track an individual's activity in an electronic system (e.g., view, print, edit)
Pending reports	Reports that have been initiated by a member of the healthcare team but not yet authenticated and may not be available for viewing by staff until completed; an EHR system will keep these documents in a pending or incomplete status

Administrative and Derived Data

There are many types of patient-identifiable data elements that are pulled from the patient's healthcare record that are not included in the legal health record or designated record set definitions. Administrative data and derived data and documents are two examples of patient-identifiable data that are used in the healthcare organization.

Administrative data are patient-identifiable data used for administrative, regulatory, healthcare operation, and payment (financial) purposes. Examples

---

[29] Sedona Conference. 2005 (September). The Sedona guidelines: Best practice guidelines and commentary for managing information & records in the electronic age. Available online at http://www.thesedonaconference.org/content/miscFiles/TSG9_05.pdf.

- Audit trails related to the EHR
- Authorization forms for release of information
- Birth and death certificate worksheets
- Correspondence concerning requests for records
- Databases containing patient information
- Event history and audit trails
- Financial and insurance forms
- Incident or patient safety reports
- Institutional review board lists
- Logs
- Notice of privacy practices acknowledgments (unless the organization chooses to classify them as part of the health record)
- Patient-identifiable data reviewed for quality assurance or utilization management
- Protocols and clinical pathways, practice guidelines, and other knowledge sources that do not imbed patient data
- Work lists and works-in-progress

Derived or administrative data are derived from the primary healthcare record and contain selected data elements to aid in the provision, support, evaluation, or advancement of patient care. Derived data and documents should be provided the same level of confidentiality as the legal health record. However, derived data should not be considered part of the health record and would not be produced in response to a court order, subpoena or request for the health record.

Derived data consist of information aggregated or summarized from patient records so that there are no means to identify patients. Examples of derived data are:

- Accreditation reports
- Anonymous patient data for research purposes
- Best-practice guidelines created from aggregate patient data
- OASIS reports
- ORYX, Quality Indicator, Quality Measure, or other reports
- Public health reports that do not contain patient-identifiable data
- Statistical reports
- Transmission reports for MDS, OASIS, and IRF PAI

APPENDIX D SOURCES

AHIMA e-HIM Work Group on the Legal Health Record. 2005 (September). Update: Guidelines for defining the legal health record for disclosure purposes. *Journal of AHIMA* 76(8): 64A-G. Available online in the AHIMA Body of Knowledge at http://www.ahima.org.

Hughes, G. 2003 (January). Defining the designated record set. *Journal of AHIMA* 74(1): 64A-D. Available online in the AHIMA Body of Knowledge at http://www.ahima. org.

Appendix E: Policy Definitions

Editor's note: this appendix contains work previously published by AHIMA.

Definitions

The following definitions may be helpful for organizations when creating the legal health record and designated record set policies. Any key terms the organization identifies should also be included in the organization's final policy.

Business record: "a recording/record made or received in conjunction with a business purpose and preserved as evidence or because the information has value. Because this information is created, received, and maintained as evidence and information by an organization or person, in pursuance of legal obligation or in the transaction of business, it must consistently deliver a full and accurate record with no gaps or additions."[30]

Data: basic facts about people, processes, measurements, and conditions represented in dates, numerical statistics, images, and symbols. An unprocessed collection or representation of raw facts, concepts, or instructions in a manner suitable for communication, interpretation, or processing by humans or automatic means.[31]

Data element: a combination of one or more data entities that forms a unit or piece of information, such as patient identifier, a diagnosis, or treatment.[32]

Electronic health record: medical information compiled in a data-gathering format for retention and transferral of protected information via secured, encrypted communication line. The information can be readily stored on an acceptable storage medium such as compact disc.[33]

Evidence: information that a fact finder may use to decide an issue. Information that makes a fact or issue before court or other hearing more or less probable.[34]

Legal health record: AHIMA defines the legal health record as "generated at or for a healthcare organization as its business record and is the record that would be released upon request. It does not affect the discoverability of other information held by the organization. The custodian of the legal health record is the health information manager in collaboration with information technology personnel. HIM professionals oversee the operational functions related to collecting, protecting, and archiving the legal health record, while information technology staff manage the technical infrastructure of the electronic health record."[35]

---

[30] AHIMA e-HIM Work Group on e-Discovery. 2006 (September). New electronic discovery civil rule. *Journal of AHIMA* 77(8): 68A-H.
[31] AHIMA e-HIM Work Group on the Legal Health Record. 2005 (September). Update: Guidelines for defining the legal health record for disclosure purposes. *Journal of AHIMA* 76(8): 64A-G.
[32] Ibid.
[33] Ibid.
[34] Ibid.
[35] Ibid.

The legal health record is a formally defined legal business record for a healthcare organization. It includes documentation of healthcare services provided to an individual in any aspect of healthcare delivery by a healthcare organization.[36],[37] The health record is individually identifiable data in any medium, collected and directly used in documenting healthcare or health status. The term also includes records of care in any health-related setting used by healthcare professionals while providing patient care services, reviewing patient data, or documenting observations, actions, or instructions.[38]

Original document: an authentic writing as opposed to a copy.[39]

Regular course of business: doing business in accordance with the normal practice of business and custom, as opposed to doing it differently because an organization may be or is being sued.[40]

Source systems: The systems in which data were originally created.

⊙ Primary source system: an information system that is part of the overall clinical information system in which documentation is most commonly first entered or generated.

⊙ Source of legal health record: the permanent storage system where the documentation for the legal health record is held.

Appendix F: Legal Health Record Sample Template

Editor's note: this appendix contains work previously published by AHIMA.

Legal Health Record Policy Template
Policy Name: The Health Record for Legal and Business Purposes
Effective Date:
Departments Affected: HIM, Information Systems, Legal Services, [any additional departments affected]
Purpose: This policy identifies the health record of [organization] for business and legal purposes and to ensure that the integrity of the health record is maintained so that it can support business and legal needs.
Scope: This policy applies to all uses and disclosures of the health record for administrative, business, or evidentiary purposes. It encompasses records that may be kept in a variety of media including, but not limited to, electronic, paper, digital images, video, and audio. It excludes those health records not normally made and kept in the regular course of the business of [organization].

---

[36] Amatayakul, M., et al. 2001 (October). Definition of the health record for legal purposes. *Journal of AHIMA* 72(9): 88A-H.

[37] AHIMA e-HIM Work Group on the Legal Health Record. 2005 (September). Update: Guidelines for defining the legal health record for disclosure purposes." *Journal of AHIMA* 76(8): 64A-G.

[38] Ibid.

[39] Ibid.

[40] Ibid.

[40] Ibid.

Note: The determining factor in whether a document is considered part of the legal health record is not where the information resides or its format, but rather how the information is used and whether it is reasonable to expect the information to be routinely released when a request for a complete health record is received. The legal health record excludes health records that are not official business records of a healthcare provider. Organizations should seek legal counsel when deciding what constitutes the organization's legal health record.

Policy: It is the policy of [organization] to create and maintain health records that, in addition to their primary intended purpose of clinical and patient care use, will also serve the business and legal needs of [organization].

It is the policy of [organization] to maintain health records that will not be compromised and will support the business and legal needs of [organization].

Routine disclosures will only include information needed to fulfill the intent of the request. It excludes information determined to not be included in the legal health record.

Responsibilities

It is the responsibility of the Health Information Management Director, working in conjunction with the Information Services Department (IS) and the Legal Department [or other appropriate departments] to:

- Maintain a matrix or other document that tracks the source, location, and media of each component of the health record. [Reference an addendum or other source where the health record information is found.]

- Identify any content that may be used in decision making and care of the patient that may be external to the organization (outside records and reports, PHRs, e-mail, etc.) that is not included as part of the legal record because it was not made or kept in the regular course of business.

- Develop, coordinate, and administer a plan that manages all information content, regardless of location or form that comprises the legal health record of [organization].

- Develop, coordinate, and administer the process of disclosure of health information.

- Develop and administer a health record retention schedule that complies with applicable regulatory and business requirements.

- Ensure appropriate access to information systems containing components of the health record

- Execute the archiving and retention schedule pursuant to the established retention schedule

- [Other responsibilities]

[Additional responsibilities for other individuals or departments]

Appendix G: Sample Designated Record Set Template

Editor's note: this appendix contains work previously published by AHIMA.

Designated Record Set Template

Policy Name: Designated Record Set Policy

Effective Date:

Departments Affected: HIM, Information Systems, Legal Services, [any additional departments affected]

Purpose: The purpose of this policy is to establish guidelines for the definition and content of the [organization] designated record set in accordance with the Health Insurance Portability and Assurance Act (HIPAA) of 1996.

Scope: This policy applies to all uses and disclosures of the health record. It encompasses records that may be kept in a variety of media including, but not limited to, electronic, paper, digital images, video, and audio. It excludes those health records not normally made and kept in the regular course of the business of [organization].

Note: The determining factor in whether a document is considered part of the designated record set is not where the information resides or its format, but rather how the information is used and whether it is reasonable to expect the information to be routinely released when a request from the individual to inspect, copy or request an amendment. The designated record set excludes health records that are not official business records of a healthcare provider. Organizations should seek legal counsel when deciding what constitutes the organization's designated record set.

Policy: To define the specific information or records that patient's may access and amend under the Health Insurance Portability and Accountability Act (HIPAA) and state privacy laws. The standards provide that individuals have the right to inspect and obtain a copy and request amendment of medical information used to make decisions about their care and billing information.

Definitions:

Designated Record Set: A group of records maintained by or for [organization] that includes the medical records and billing records about individuals that is used in whole or part by or for [organization] to make decisions about individuals. The term record is defined as any item, collection, or grouping of information that includes protected health information and is maintained, collected, used, or disseminated by or for [organization].

Includes:

- Legal medical record (refer to your organization's Legal Health Record Policy)
- Patient-specific claim information such as encounter forms, claims submitted, account balances, payment agreements, ABN letters, notice of noncoverage letters, etc.

- Outside facility or provider records used in whole or in part by [organization] to make decisions about individuals
- Patient-submitted documentation and referral letters
- Other patient-specific information such as consents and authorizations

Excludes:

- Administrative data, which is patient-identifiable and used for administrative, regulatory, or other healthcare operations, such as event history/audit trails, data used for quality assurance or utilization management, data prepared in anticipation of legal action, etc.
- Derived data stored in aggregate or summarized which is not patient-identifiable, such as data used for accreditation reports, research data, statistical reports, best practice guidelines, etc.
- Psychotherapy notes maintained separate from the rest of the patient's medical record
- Patient information created as part of a research study to which the patient has temporarily waived right to access
- Records that have been destroyed because they have exceeded their required retention period or because they have been rendered unusable due to fire, flood, or other circumstances
- Information that is subject to a legal privilege such as peer review or attorney/client privilege

Excluded from designated record set but may be disclosed with appropriate authorization:

- Source data such as radiology films, videos, photographs, slides, EKG strips, fetal monitor strips, etc., when available

Responsibilities

It is the responsibility of the Health Information Management Director, working in conjunction with the Information Services Department (IS) and the Legal Department [or other appropriate departments] to:

- Maintain a matrix or other document that tracks the source, location, and media of each component of the health record [reference an addendum or other source where the health record information is found]
- Identify any content that may be used in decision making and care of the patient that may be external to the organization (outside records and reports, PHRs, e-mail, etc.) that is not included as part of the legal record because it was not made or kept in the regular course of business
- Develop, coordinate, and administer a plan that manages all information content, regardless of location or form that comprises the legal health record of [organization]

- Develop, coordinate, and administer the process of inspecting, copying, and amending health information
- Develop and administer a health record retention schedule that complies with applicable regulatory and business requirements
- Ensure appropriate access to information systems containing components of the health record
- Execute the archiving and retention schedule pursuant to the established retention schedule
- [Other responsibilities]

[Additional responsibilities for other individuals or departments]

REFERENCES

American Health Information Management Association. 2010 (May). Guidance for clinical documentation improvement programs. *Journal of AHIMA* 81(5): expanded web version. Available online in the AHIMA Body of Knowledge at http://www.ahima.org.

Centers for Medicare and Medicaid Services, Department of Health and Human Services. Title 42 Public Health. Chapter IV, Subchapter G Standards and Certification. Part 482 Conditions of Participation for Hospitals, Subpart C Basic Hospital Functions. Section 482.24 Condition of Participation: Medical Record Services. Available online at http://cfr.vlex.com/vid/482-condition-participation-record-19811382#ixzz13345288z.

Department of Health and Human Services. 2002 (August 14). Standards for Privacy of Individually Identifiable Health Information; Final Rule. 45 CFR Parts 160 and 164. *Federal Register* 67, no. 157. Available online at http://aspe.hhs.gov/admnsimp/final/pvcguide1.htm.

Joint Commission. The Joint Commission Standards. Available online at http://www.jointcommission.org/Standards.

NCHICA Designated Record Sets Work Group and Privacy and Confidentiality Focus Group. 2002 (August 16). Guidance for Identifying Designated Record Sets under HIPAA. Available online at http://www.nchica.org/HIPAA Resources/Samples/DesRecSets.pdf.

Servais, C. E. 2008. *The Legal Health Record*. Chicago, IL: AHIMA.

Warner, D. 2010 (March). Evaluating alerts and triggers: Determining whether alerts and triggers are part of the legal health record. *Journal of AHIMA* 81(3): 40-41. Available online in the AHIMA Body of Knowledge at http://www.ahima.org.

ACKNOWLEDGMENTS

Cecilia Backman, MBA, RHIA, CPHQ

Angela Dinh, MHA, RHIA, CHPS

Denise Dunyak, MS, RHIA

Suzy Johnson, MS, RHIA

Nicole Miller, RHIA

Mary Stanfill, MBI, RHIA, CCS,
  CCS-P, FAHIMA

Allison Viola, MBA, RHIA

The information contained in this practice brief reflects the consensus opinion of the professionals who developed it. It has not been validated through scientific research.

MCKESSON

Case Study

....

Organization

Community Hospital of the Monterey Peninsula Monterey, Calif.

- Nonprofit organization

- 325 physicians; 15 locations including main hospital, outpatient facilities, hospice, laboratories and offices

Solution Spotlight

- McKesson Business Folder™

- McKesson Patient Folder™

Critical Issues

- Inefficient paper-based processes

- Difficulty accessing the patients' complete medical record

- Chart deficiencies

- Denied claims due to incomplete documentation

- High A/R days and operational expenses

- Regulatory compliance

Results

- Gained the ability to manage the legal medical record and coding processes from one location

- Reduced chart deficiencies and achieved 100% physician utilization

- Reduced DNFB patient accounts from six days to 2.5 days

- Eliminated four FTEs

- Reduced supply costs by $30,600 per year

- Enabled regulatory compliance

Community Hospital of the Monterey Peninsula Gains Efficiencies and Reduces Operating Expenses with HIM Solutions

Community Hospital of the Monterey Peninsula (CHOMP), a nonprofit healthcare provider in Monterey, Calif., has grown and evolved in direct response to the changing healthcare needs of the people it serves. When it became apparent that paper-based processes were inhibiting access to critical patient information, delaying reimbursement and compromising regulatory compliance, the organization took action. CHOMP implemented a health information management (HIM) solution from McKesson. Now the complete medical record can be accessed electronically from one location. As a result, reimbursement is quicker, operational expenses have decreased, chart deficiencies are low and regulatory compliance is easier.

Challenges

CHOMP had faced significant challenges managing paper charts. Physician deficiency rates continued to increase, and charts were piled high in the health information management (HIM) department. Because of the many file cabinets required to store the charts, there was little room for HIM staff. Accounts receivable

days were high, and claims were denied due to incomplete documentation. Retrieving the required documentation often took more than three days, delaying payment to the hospital.

Answers

CHOMP went live with McKesson Patient Folder™ to optimize HIM processes, improve physicians' access to patient information and enable management of the complete legal medical record. The solution helped physicians to complete chart deficiencies online and streamlined HIM processes.

When CHOMP went live with Sunrise XA™ two years later, McKesson Patient Folder easily integrated with the clinical system to enable physicians to access critical patient information. As a result, physicians can access deficiency worklists, patient information from all encounters, cardiopulmonary and radiology reports, and wound photos managed in McKesson Patient Folder directly from the physician view in the clinical system. All patient and physician context is transferred across the system, eliminating the need for multiple sign-ons or patient search.

"Managing the legal medical record and coding processes for multiple departments from a single location has significantly improved operational efficiencies and reduced costs across the organization."

— *Madelyn Burke, RHIA Director, Health Information Management Community Hospital of the Monterey Peninsula*

McKesson Technology Solutions
5995 Windward Parkway
Alpharetta, GA 30005

www.mckesson.com

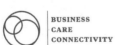

BUSINESS
CARE
CONNECTIVITY

CHOMP also implemented McKesson Business Folder™ in the business department to expedite claims resolution and reduce documentation-related denials.

Results

"Managing the legal medical record and coding processes for multiple departments from a single location has significantly improved operational efficiencies and reduced costs across the organization," states Madelyn Burke, RHIA, director, Health Information Management, CHOMP. "Equally important, the ability to control all of this information in a single system enables us to comply with HIPAA and The Joint Commission standards."

Within six months of implementing McKesson Patient Folder, CHOMP reduced DNFB (days not final billed) patient accounts from six days to 2.5 days, resulting in a one-time cash benefit of $4,379,354 in today's dollars. The HIM department reduced full-time equivalents (FTEs) by four and eliminated the night shift. As a result, CHOMP saved $222,500 per year in staff expenses.

Claims are resolved faster because documentation is readily available. The billing department now provides history and physical or discharge summaries in response to insurance company requests within a day, making claims resolution faster and cash flow stronger.

The elimination of paper records and off-site storage enabled CHOMP to reduce supply costs by more than $30,600 per year, enabling the organization to save more than $214,000 since implementing the solution. Also, abandoning filing cabinets allowed HIM staff to be centralized in one area and freed space for hospital engineers.

CHOMP achieved 100% physician utilization, with more than 350 physicians using the system. Satisfaction among physicians significantly improved because they can access all patient information and complete deficiencies online, anywhere and anytime. Emergency room documents are available for viewing online within six hours, and inpatient and outpatient documents are available within 24 hours of patient discharge.

Simple and intuitive, user-configurable workflows have enabled CHOMP to create new automated processes to address specific business needs. Additionally, CHOMP is confident that McKesson Patient Folder will enable it to address current industry challenges.

"McKesson Patient Folder provides everything we need to manage the RAC audit process, including workflow and electronic chart release," states Burke. "We can also include InterQual® letters and official documentation validating the appropriateness of physician decisions within the patient's record and easily send it all together from the beginning. Now that's an efficient system."

MᶜKESSON

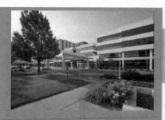

CHARTMAXX CUSTOMER
Bryan Medical Center
Lincoln, Nebraska

QUICK FACTS
• HealthGrades: Ranked top 5% in the nation for overall orthopedics
• Two different facilities: West and East Campuses
• Total Beds: 672
• Staff: 3,500+
• Admissions: 33,000
• CIS: Siemens INVISION® (March 2010 – Go Live with Siemens Soarian®)
• Physician Portal: Developed in house

RESULTS ACHIEVED
• Reduced Health Information Management operating budget by 40% the first year.
• Reduced chart delinquencies by 80%.
• Increased coding productivity by 33%.
• Decreased Release of Information turnaround time by 250%.
• Recovered $3.9 million in revenue by reducing the time to code charts.
• Improved ease of compliance with HIPAA and Joint Commission regulations and reduced audit time from 3-5 days to 3-5 hours.

ChartMaxx Success Profile

Bryan Medical Center   ChartMaxx®

Bryan is one medical center at two locations, providing a comprehensive range of healthcare services, resources, state-of-the-art facilities and access to over 3,500 professionals who deliver high quality care to more than 33,000 patients a year.

Over the years, Bryan Medical Center has been nationally recognized as a top hospital in the country by independent rating companies Solucient and HealthGrades, and was selected in 2013 as Top 50 Cardiovascular Hospital by Truven Health Analytics and Best Performer Award in Discharge Preparedness from Avatar International.

SITUATION:
Two Systems to One - Hindered by Multiple Processes and Impacting Billing Processes

The top priority for Bryan Medical Center was to integrate the two disparate medical records systems used at its West and East campuses using a comprehensive, enterprise-wide, electronic medical record solution. Not only was each campus using different systems, they were operating with unique chart management policies and procedures resulting in complication, confusion and extra costs.

The medical staff was also challenged by labor-intensive and unproductive paper chart processes impeding the billing process. Coders waited for days to code the chart which often lacked vital information to complete work. Physicians had difficulty accessing patient charts, resulting in sporadic dictation and delays in final approval. These manual processes resulted in a chart delinquency rate of 31%. Given the multiple processes and systems, preparation for audit reviews took 3-5 days. Often patient charts had to be manually located, pulled and verified – a time consuming and inefficient process.

"Our labor-intensive process of locating records for one patient in two hospital campuses in a timely manner had gotten out of control," says Nadene Powell, RHIA, Health Information Management (HIM) Manager, Imaging Center. "We needed to find a better way to provide our physicians and staff with easy access to patient information and merge our processes across our continuum of care to help physicians and staff complete charts."

Quest Diagnostics

> "The ability to pull records from my office when I have a minute means I don't have to make a trip to the hospital. Plus, 'anywhere' access to historical records is helpful when admitting a patient."
>
> **Michael Myers, M.D.**
> **MDLMEF Family Practice Center**

> "We have a stable staff and job satisfaction is high because of our ability to realize success on a daily basis. Charts can now be automatically pulled and sent electronically for audit review without an auditor even stepping into our hospital. We know staff and physician satisfaction translates to better care for patients."
>
> **Karen Kurbis, RHIA, Corporate Compliance & Research.**

> "We needed to have the right information at the right time in the right format to take care of patients optimally. The more reliable and available the information, the better care we can provide and we needed an EHR system that could help us deliver it."
>
> **Lois Givens, RHIA, Director of HIM**

ChartMaxx ECM with an advanced Business Process Management platform is aimed at helping hospitals solve critical IT priorities, improving the patient experience, enabling workflow efficiency and providing a greater return on investment.

ChartMaxx enables hospitals with a fast deployment and short time-to-value to create highly efficient workflow processes. This uniquely fast, easy and customized path will help your organization connect systems, information, people and processes together in order to provide timely access to focused and actionable information.

ChartMaxx Success Profile

ChartMaxx®

SOLUTION:
One System. . .One Process. . .Numerous Benefits.

Employing ChartMaxx at the East and West campuses simultaneously using a "big bang" approach, Bryan realized immediate results and a continued, steady, measurable improvement in performance. ChartMaxx provided the electronic enterprise-wide solution to integrate all of Bryan hospital facilities into one unified and comprehensive health record process – providing instant, concurrent chart access and streamlining cumbersome paper-based manual processes.

ChartMaxx consolidated the campus systems into one streamlined, cohesive and multifunctional electronic system improving workflows and reducing costs.

RESULTS

ChartMaxx anytime, anywhere access allowed physicians to easily review and sign patient charts, lowering the hospital's chart delinquency rate from 31% down to 6%. Reduced time for coding resulted in an additional $3.9 million in increased revenue the first year.

In addition to helping to improve patient care throughout the enterprise and increasing revenue, ChartMaxx also enhanced productivity and delivered on other metrics – including a reduction in HIM operating costs of more than 40% the first year.

Release of Information also saw immediate results – turnaround time decreased from 11 days to 2 days. Additionally, charts for audits are now easily located and sent out electronically on the same day of the request.

For HIM, the ability to simultaneously review accurate and timely patient charts improved the chart completion process, resulting in a 33% increase in coder productivity. One sure indication of success – employee turnover among coders has become nonexistent

The benefits of ChartMaxx have extended to improving regulatory compliance. By using the ChartMaxx robust security features, the HIM department maintains greater control over medical records and better safeguarding against unauthorized access to confidential patient information while maintaining an account of disclosures. HIPAA guidelines and Joint Commission regulations are easily and quickly met and audits that once took 3-5 days to conduct now take 3-5 hours to complete.

In addition to the patient-centric model, the HIM team is using the ChartMaxx "electronic file cabinet" functionality to manage forms and Forms Committee documentation. The HIM department has benefited so much that it is promoting the use of the electronic file cabinet feature to other departments including Medical Staff Affairs for physician files, Human Resources for employee files and Public Relations for publications and meeting minutes.

ChartMaxx Client Success Study—Bryan Medical Center, 2013 Quest Diagnostics Incorporated

CASE STUDY

SARASOTA MEMORIAL HEALTH CARE SYSTEM: ONE DOOR TO THE ELECTRONIC HEALTH RECORD

INTEGRATING PAPER AND ELECTRONIC INFORMATION INTO A COMPREHENSIVE PATIENT "STORY OF CARE"

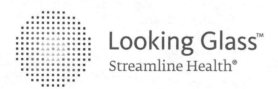

Enterprise Content Management

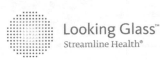

ONE DOOR TO THE ELECTRONIC HEALTH RECORD

Is it electronic medical record or electronic health record? Is it a "paperless" EMR or a "hybrid"? Is it a legal health record and if so, what must that include? What do the new Certification Commission for Healthcare Information Technology (CCHIT) terms - "certified" and "qualified" – mean to an organization?

Sarasota Memorial Health Care System (SMHCS) pursued a vision rather than a label: "One Door to the Electronic Health Record." They challenged themselves to improve quality and safety of patient care, ease the burden on physicians by providing them with complete patient record access and strengthen outcomes with optimized information access. The directive was access to and completion of the entire medical record from one user interface regardless of the origination of information – paper or electronic, internal or external.

Through creation of a fully integrated EMR incorporating the "ScanDocs" document management tab, SMHCS has realized a one-time cash flow boost of $1 million dollars and reduced operating expenses by $500,000 per year. Moreover, physicians and their staffs are happier and patient safety is improved because the entire patient story is online and accessible from anywhere; care decisions are fully informed and timelier.

Now that physicians no longer go to medical records for chart completion, SMHCS is considering the recovery and repurposing of premium floor space by moving non-revenue generating departments off-site.

"We initially looked at HIM departmental systems but we wanted one place for the physicians to go. Everything needs to be accessible through the EMR. We now have a decade of EMR data online"

Denis Baker, Chief Information Officer,
Sarasota Memorial Health Care System

Streamline Health enhanced SMHCS's vision by emphasizing document management as a critical enterprise-wide workflow solution rather than a departmental application. Streamline Health offered a distinct approach of integrated vs. interfaced so document management becomes a seamless component of the clinical system with a common user interface and immediate information access.

THE JOURNEY TO A COMPLETE PATIENT STORY OF CARE

Like all worthy endeavors, creating the holistic patient story of care occurred in several stages:

Phase I: Image Enabling Key Documents

Phase II: The ScanDocs Tab

Phase III: Online Chart Completion

PHASE I: IMAGE ENABLING KEY DOCUMENTS

The first stage of the journey began by constructing an integrated document selection tree within Sunrise Clinical Manager (SCM) – including transcribed documents, free text notes, nursing flow sheets and wound care images held in the document management system. SMHCS focused on image enabling the most requested documents:

- Continuity of Care
  - EKGs
  - Emergency Room documentation
  - History and Physical
  - Surgical documentation
- Patient Identification and Fraud Prevention
  - Driver's Licenses
  - Insurance Cards
- Patient Safety
  - Advance Directives
  - Living Wills
  - Power of Attorney

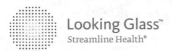
Looking Glass™
Streamline Health®

PHASE II: THE SCANDOCS TAB

The second stage created direct access to all the documents residing in the document management system from within the SCM user interface. The tab is configurable so SMHCS conducted a "name that tab" contest; ScanDocs was selected as the winner. Critical development in phase two involved ease of access; both patient context and user security needed to pass from SCM to Streamline Health's enterprise content management (ECM) solution to prevent duplicate patient look up or redundant authentication. Document viewing inherits role based security so if a user is restricted from access to a certain document (e.g. psychiatric documents) then that specific document is view-locked.

PHASE III: ONLINE CHART COMPLETION

The final phase implemented a chart completion inbox in the ScanDocs tab along with chart deficiency reporting. This last important step allowed SMHCS to migrate to online chart completion from within the EMR. Because this was a significant change to physician workflow, a roll-out campaign was launched. A pre-live raffle enticed physicians to close out all open paper record deficiencies with a raffle ticket offered for each completion. Several "Snippets" – one page training flyers – communicated the new workflow which was so intuitive that a 10 minute orientation available in the physician's lounge was sufficient for introductory training.

Doctors now had on-line chart completion including signature, dictation, and annotation in an intuitive email inbox paradigm. No more trips to the Health Information Management (HIM) Department were necessary and they gained remote access for chart completion.

For the HIM department, it was a total transition from traditional paper record processing to performing all chart deficiency analysis and reporting online.

And SMHCS had achieved One Door to the Electronic Health Record.

"Accessibility is critical: the combination of EMR/CPOE/Streamline Health in one place is tremendous. I can respond to anything from work, home, or out of town – I review EKGs and pre-op clearance online. And I never go to medical records anymore because I see all my chart deficiencies online, I can complete and sign charts from anywhere."

James Florica, MD, Gynecological Oncologist, Sarasota Memorial Health Care System

THE PHYSICIAN'S DOOR

With the go-live of on-line chart completion, physicians now had One Door to the entire patient story. From the SCM user interface, physicians access electronic medical records, sign orders and transcribed reports, get results, view scanned documents and sign/annotate documents... anytime, anywhere

Deficiency reporting creates a quick view of open chart items for physicians. Physicians can quickly filter items as desired for immediate action. Results are automatically updated in the ScanDocs inbox and in the completion dashboard.

INTEGRATING ENTERPRISE CONTENT MANAGEMENT WITH SUNRISE CLINICAL MANAGER

Helios™

Helios is the integration toolkit – based on the Microsoft .NET framework – used to extend Sunrise Clinical Manager functionality. Early in development, Streamline Health worked directly with SCM developers, who provided guidance and support on the architectural approach for using Helios to develop the integration.

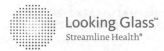

Looking Glass™
Streamline Health®

Application-to-Application Messaging

SMHCS required no duplication of information. All image enabled documents are available for viewing or printing from within SCM via a document pointer that creates links within the SCM user interface.

After a document is created within Streamline's ECM, a customizable pointer is sent to SCM via the Helios API with the following fields:

- Medical Record Number
- Account Number
- Document Sequence Number
- Document Type
- Entity ID

Patient Context and User Authentication

SMHCS required seamless physician access between SCM and Streamline's ECM. Patient context is set in SCM and automatically synchronized in the ScanDocs tab. Likewise, single sign-on is supported: the user authenticates once to SCM and those credentials are accepted by the document management environment. SMHCS elected to enable password entry as the physicians' method of electronically signing documents.

OUTCOMES

Below is a summary of SMHCS outcomes and improvements from the integration of Streamline Health's document management solution with SCM. We share these outcomes as potential benchmarks for your organization.

Benefits Benchmark Scorecard	Sarasota Memorial Outcomes
Financial Metric Improvements	
Net A/R Days	14%
Discharged Not Final Coded	23%
Discharged Not Final Billed	7%
Cost per Unit of Service	14%
Management to Staff Ratio	29%
FTE Reduction	9%
Physician Value	
Remote completion of ALL medical records ($75/day/400 physicians)	$1.5 million per year
Real time notification of incomplete records	Yes
Electronically EDIT & SIGN transcribed reports	Yes
Electronically ANNOTATE & SIGN paper records	Yes
Medical Records Savings	
Elimination of Record Supplies	$10,000 per year
Analysis & Retrieval Costs	$220,000 per year
Storage & Archival Media Costs	$180,000 per year
Contract coder travel expense reduction	$76,500 per year
Other Benefits	
Re-purpose prime real estate	Yes
Meet regulatory and accreditation requirements	Yes
Electronic Legal Health Record	Yes
One view to complete patient story of care	Yes

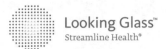

ADDITIONAL OUTCOMES

Anesthesiology Department

- Online records including outside studies permit trending, not guessing
- Online preoperative clearance helps patient safety and risk management

Health Information Management Department

- Increased productivity and opportunity to cross-train due to system efficiency
- Happier interactions with physician community
- Chart flow from ambulatory improved
- Online record facilitates Joint Commission auditing and reporting
- Release of information is substantially more efficient
- Ability to recruit coders anywhere with remote access
- Paper records destroyed 7 days after scanning and QA
- Fewer record pulls (pre-2006 records only); all reviews occur in SCM/ScanDocs

FolderAnyWare functionality allows non-clinical departments to access scanned documents

The following departments utilize the production system:

- Cancer Registry
- Clinical Systems Analyst Group
- Clinical Systems – Financial Business Systems Group
- Clinical Systems – AMPFM Group
- Corporate Finance Payroll
- HIM – Forms Committee
- HIM – Administrative
- HIM – Coding
- Human Resources
- Managed Care
- Patient Financial Services – Lockbox Images
- Patient Financial Services – Administration
- Revenue Cycle Management
- Risk Management
- SMHCS Physician Services

"By integrating comprehensive documentation workflow into Sunrise Clinical Manager, Sarasota Memorial Health Care System made major strides towards supporting the clinician 'Thoughtflow™' process – presenting actionable information when and where it's needed to enhance clinician assessment and decision-making."

Sam Bierstock, MD, BSEE
Founder, Champions in Healthcare, LLC, Former VP of Medical Affairs, Eclipsys Corporation

CONCLUSION

From an RFP to a final product implementation, SMHCS and Streamline Health created a deep integration of paper documents, record management, and online chart completion within Sunrise Clinical Manager. Together they achieved an unprecedented enterprise workflow for the complete electronic health record in a single user interface with astounding results:

- Increased patient safety
- Improved quality of care
- Dramatic gains in physician and staff satisfaction
- A one million dollar one-time cash flow boost
- $500,000 annual operating expense reduction
- And the opportunity to repurpose prime real estate by moving non-revenue generating departments off-site

Every organization takes a risk – in time, money, resources and opportunity cost – when they pursue a complex integration project. The deep integration of Streamline's ECM solution with Sunrise Clinical Manager pioneered by Sarasota Memorial Health Care System substantially mitigates the risk for any SCM client seeking the benefits of enterprise document management.

Index